All About Having A Baby

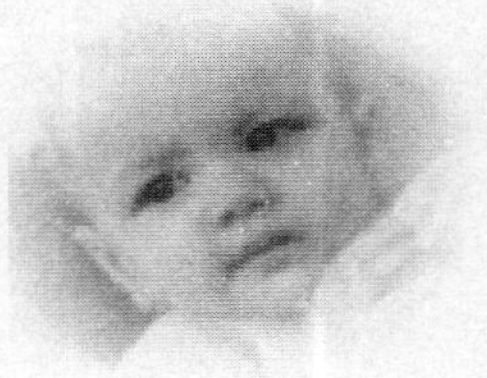

A Step-by-Step Guide On Pregnancy and Baby Care

Dr. Yatish Agarwal
Rekha Agarwal

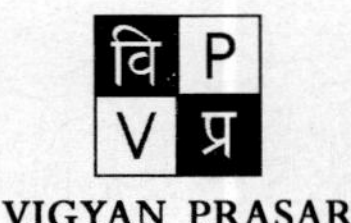

VIGYAN PRASAR

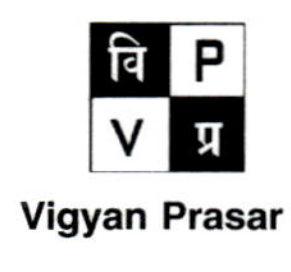

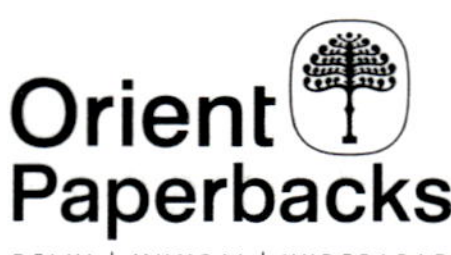

ISBN : 81-222-0430-9

First Edition 2002
Reprint 2004
Reprint 2006

Published by :
Vigyan Prasar
A-50, Institutional Area, Sector 62,
Noida - 201307 U.P.
Phone : 0120-2404430, 0120-2404439
Fax : 0120-2404437
E-mail : info@vigyanprasar.gov.org

Editor :
Arundhti Bhanot

Design & Illustrations:
Narendra

Reviewer :
Dr. Pinkee Saxena,
Safdarjung Hospital, New Delhi- 110 029

Text typeset in 14pt. Perpetua &
headings in 16 pt. Folia BdCnBT
by Chandramurari Prasad

Multi Colour Services
S-39, Okhla Indl.Area, Phase-II,
New Delhi-110020

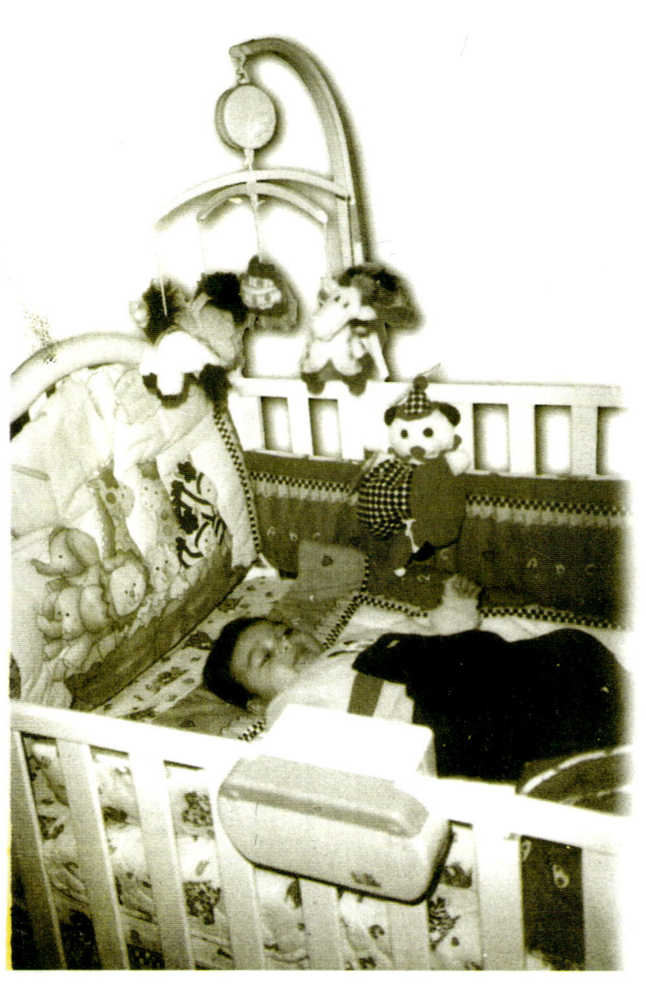

About the Authors

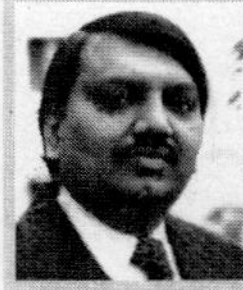

Yatish Agarwal (MBBS, MD, DSc)

Dr. Yatish Agarwal is a noted physician, writer and health columnist. His popular books, essays, articles, columns, radio broadcasts and TV serials and chat shows on the net have spread his message of good health and simple, sensible living to millions of people. Several of his books are bestsellers and now available in many languages. His columns Medibyte, You Ask We Answer and Body Talk in the leading national daily Hindustan Times and Swasthya Suljhan in the leading-most women's magazine Grihshobha are immensely popular. A Doctor of Medicine from the University of Delhi, Dr. Agarwal has been a recipient of the Atmaram Samman (1999), NCSTC National Science Award (1999), Meghnad Saha Award (1991, '92 & '93), National Excellence Award (1992-93) and Ministry of Health's National Award (1994, '95, '97). Dr. Agarwal works at New Delhi's Safdarjung Hospital. He has in the past been associated with the Vallabhbhai Patel Chest Institute, New Delhi, Rajan Babu Tuberculosis Hospital, New Delhi, and also the National Cancer Centre Hospital, Tokyo.

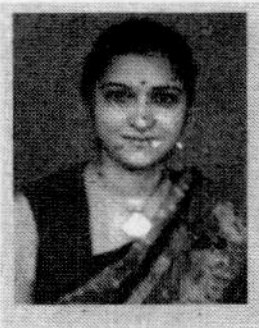

Rekha Agarwal (BSc, MA, PG Dip in Journalism)

Rekha Agarwal is a noted writer, broadcaster and editor. Her previous works include The Story of Blood, Khalifa Ki Pagdi and Nari Vigyan. Her stories and articles have been published in several leading literary journals and national dailies. Many of her works have also been translated into Oriya and Bengali. A recipient of the Hindi Akademi Award (1985) and Ministry Of Health's National Award (1997), she works as an editor with the National Council of Educational Research & Training, New Delhi.

Designer

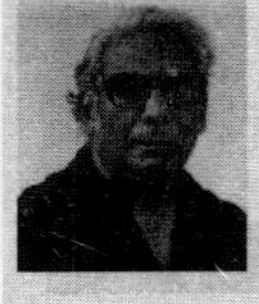

Narendra

A graphic designer of international renown, Narendra is best known for his seminal work in symbols and logos. An awardee of Jawahar Lal Nehru Fellowship(1973) and Sahitya Kala Parishad Samman(1993), he has held several one man shows in India and some of the best known art galleries in Europe. He has been the logo designer for Pierre Cardin, Paris; Asia 72; Maharja Ranjeet Singh Trust; Jahr Teller (1975); and Energie Teller Rosenthal (1979).

Other popular titles by the author

- Bodytalk
- Heart Care
- The Story of Blood

In Hindi

- Khile Matritva Goonje Kilkariyan
- Diabetes Ke Saath Jeenay Ki Raha
- Hridaya Rog
- Swasthya Ke 300 Sawal
- Jatil Rog Saral Upchar
- Pait Ke Rog
- Rog Nirog
- Sabke liye Swasthya
- Nari Vigyan
- Netra Rog
- Dampatya Vigyan
- Pyar Ke Moti
- Mann Ke Rog
- Hridaya Rog Se Cancer Tak
- Tan Mann Sadhey Sab Sadhey

Children's books

- First Aid
- Rakta Ki Kahani
- Chikitsa Vigyan Ki Kahaniyan
- Shalya Chikitsa Ki Kahani
- Nari Sharir Ka Vyakaran

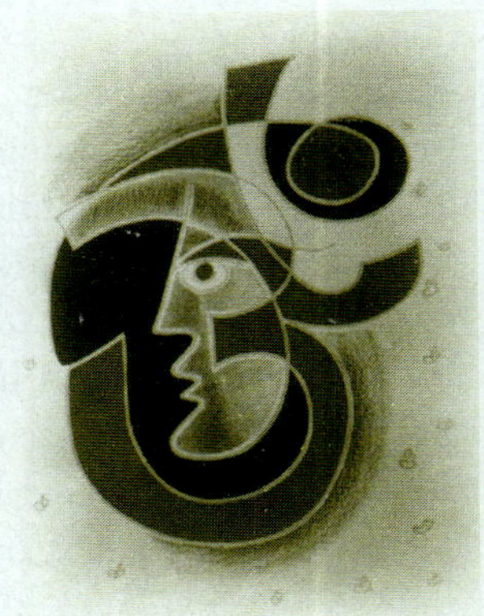

Without you I don't exist
without me You are unmanifest

To my parents Adarsh & Sat Prakash
who gave me life,
the will to know,
...and taught me
the joy of sharing.

Preface

The birth of a baby is one of the most joyful moments in one's life. It is a sacred and fulfilling experience, which changes one's whole outlook on life. A baby is a symbol of all that's beautiful, precious, and most wonderful in life. The birth of a baby in a happy, healthy family means that the bond between husband and wife has come of age. Together you create a new human being who embodies a part of each of you—your bodies, minds, and spirits, and is in a true sense, your own vision of yourselves carrying on your love and work and life into the future.

The groundwork for good parenting must begin the moment you decide upon having a baby. That is the time to take stock and make a few preparations. To set the ball rolling, you must know the rules and nuances of human plan of reproduction for your baby's safety and good health.

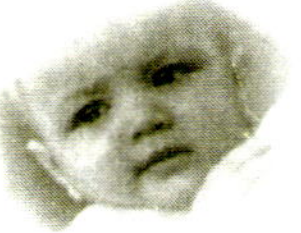

The most joyful moments.... in one's life

The moment conception occurs, the mother takes the responsibility of nurturing the seed of life. Bit by bit, cell-by-cell, perfused by her arteries the tiny fertilised egg grows into a complete baby! A single cell grows and matures into billions of cells; still each baby is unique. Only a mother can feel the tug of this special bond, only she can feel the pride of her creation. By giving birth, she ensures life's continuation.

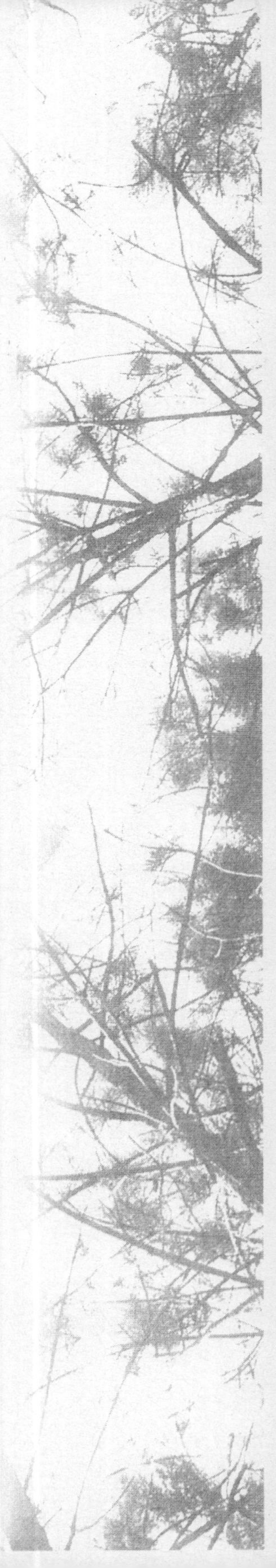

The 40 weeks or so of toil is crossed by some remarkable changes. Most women are lucky and have a fairly smooth pregnancy. However, 15 per cent pregnancies do not do well and terminate in an abortion. Again, there are times when a pregnancy gets mired in complications and requires deft handling for a satisfactory outcome.

Finally, the big day arrives. You take up a new role. Bringing up that helpless bundle of life has both its rewards and punishment. The sleepless nights, the splitting headaches are salved when the baby smiles or when those tiny fingers clasp yours. Knowing the simple rules of baby care prepares you for the tasks that lie ahead.

This book packs the present-day modern knowledge about conceiving, carrying and caring of your baby without renouncing the wisdom of old. It sifts facts from myths and fulfils the role of a friend who has the answers to most of your questions. But in no case does it pretend to be a substitute for the practical wisdom of an obstetrician who must take on the spot decisions based on the immediate evidence available to her. Make the best use of this work in this light.

Yatish Agarwal
Rekha Agarwal

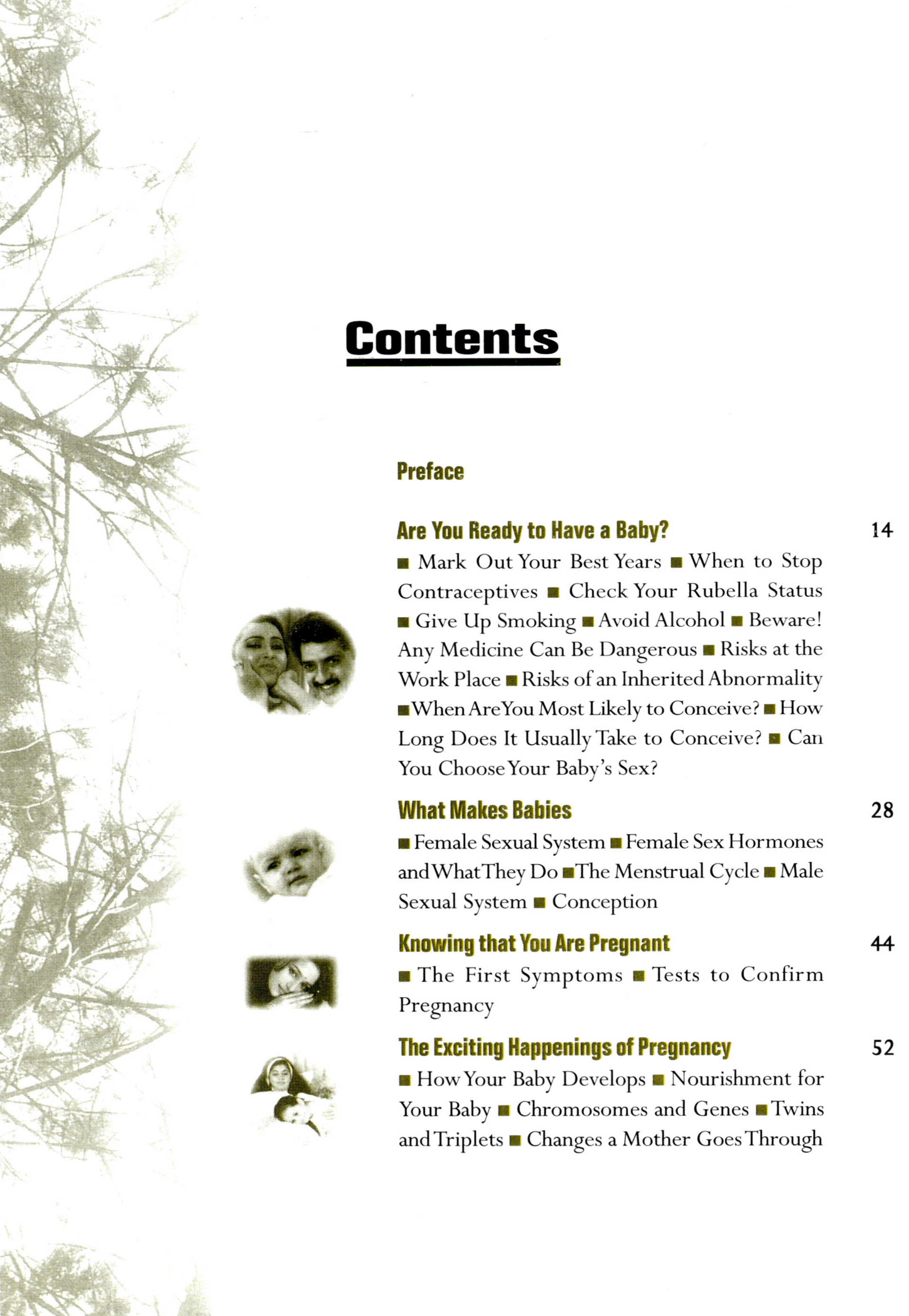

Contents

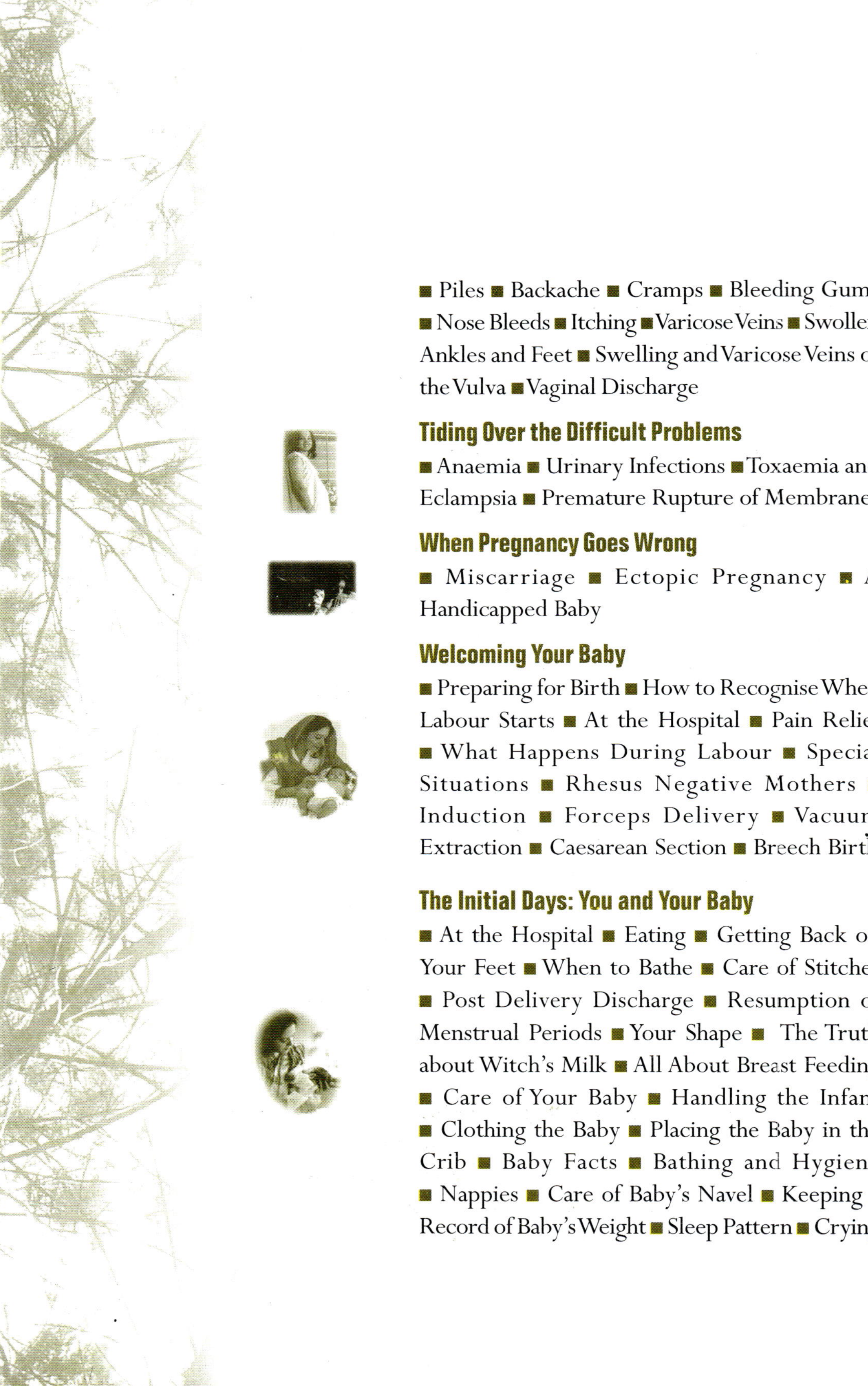

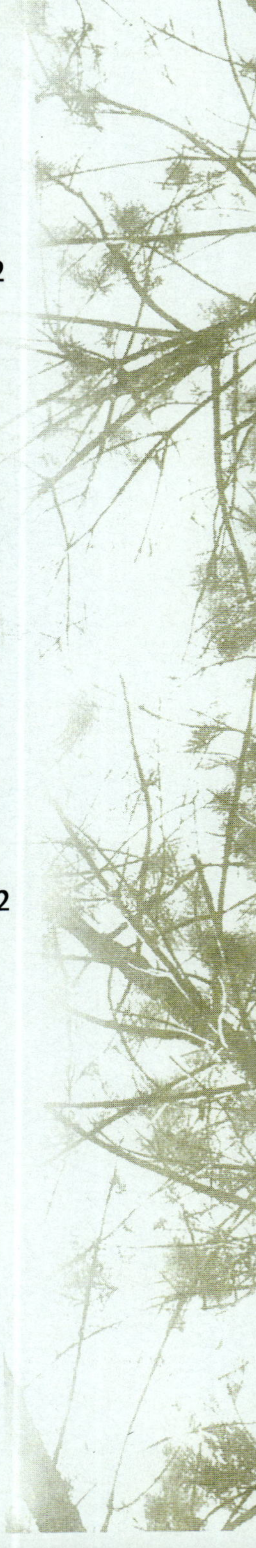

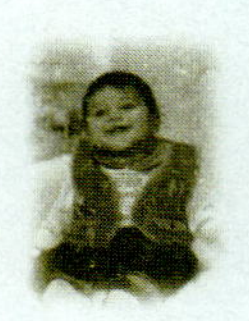

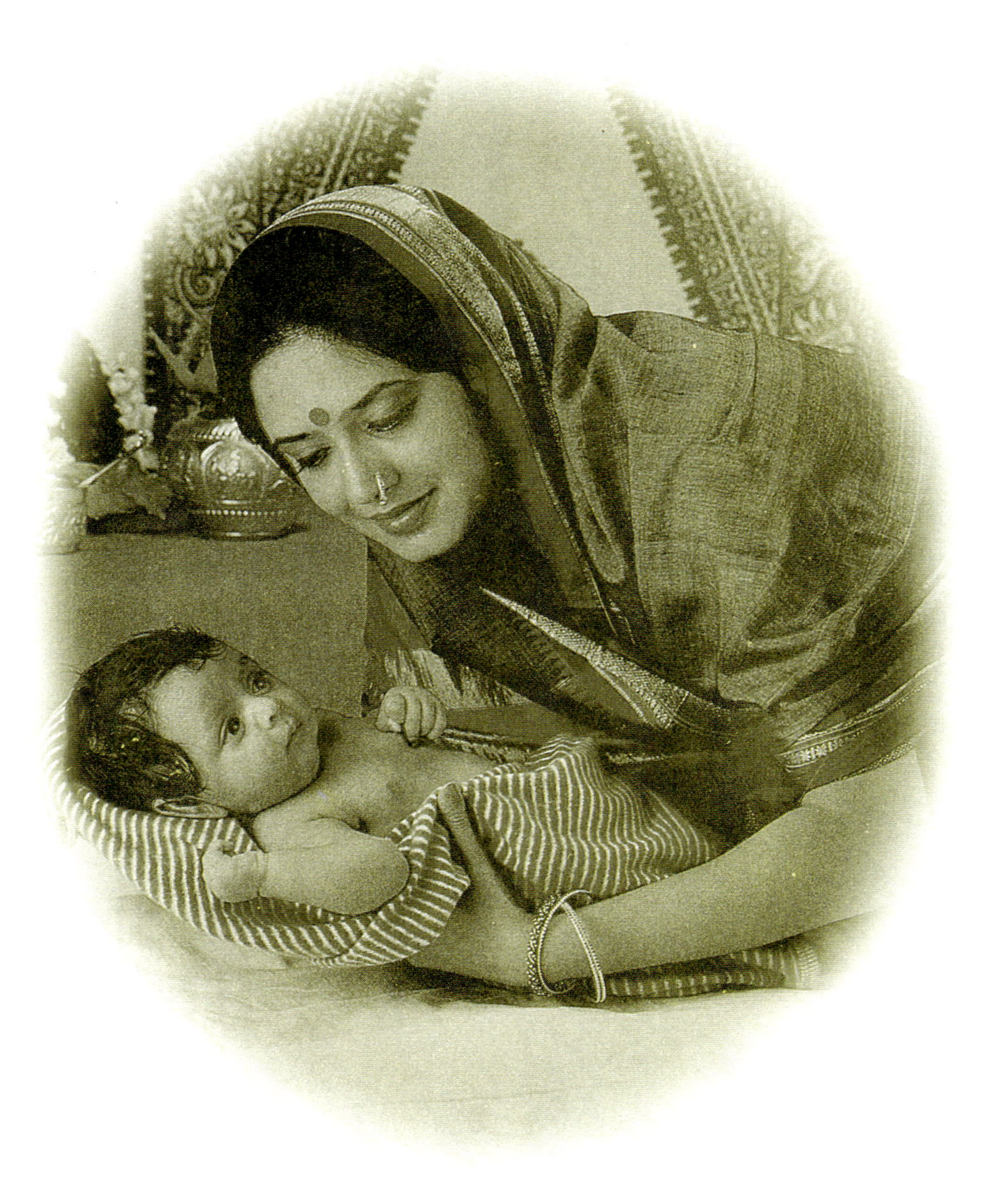

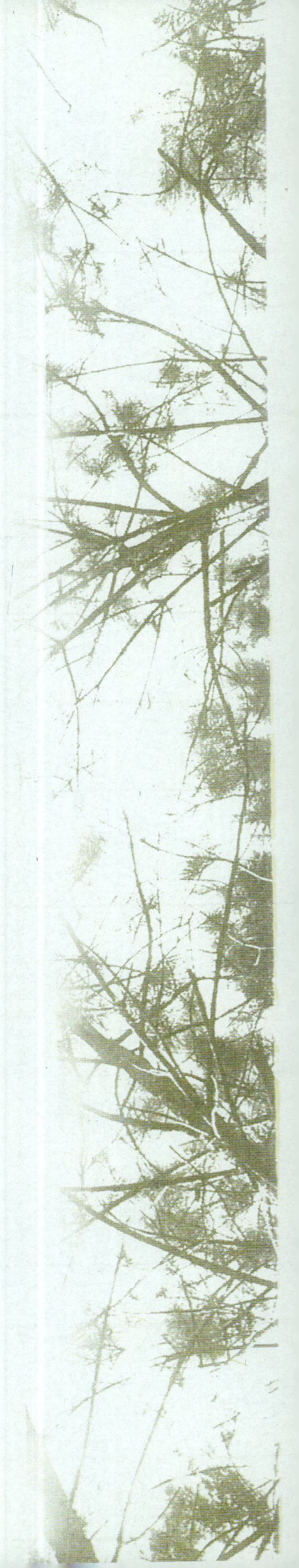

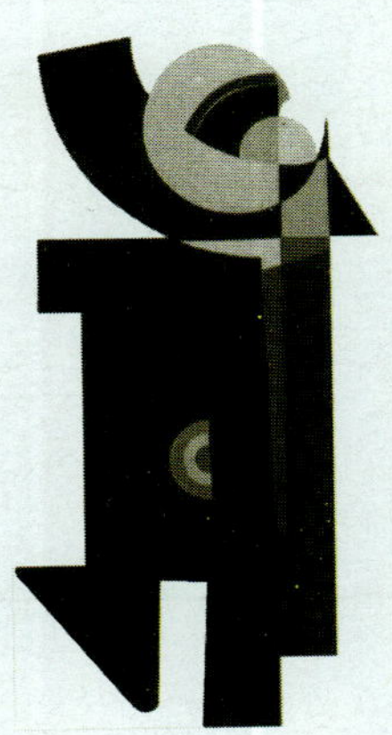

God could not be everywhere
and therefore he made mothers.

-Jewish proverb

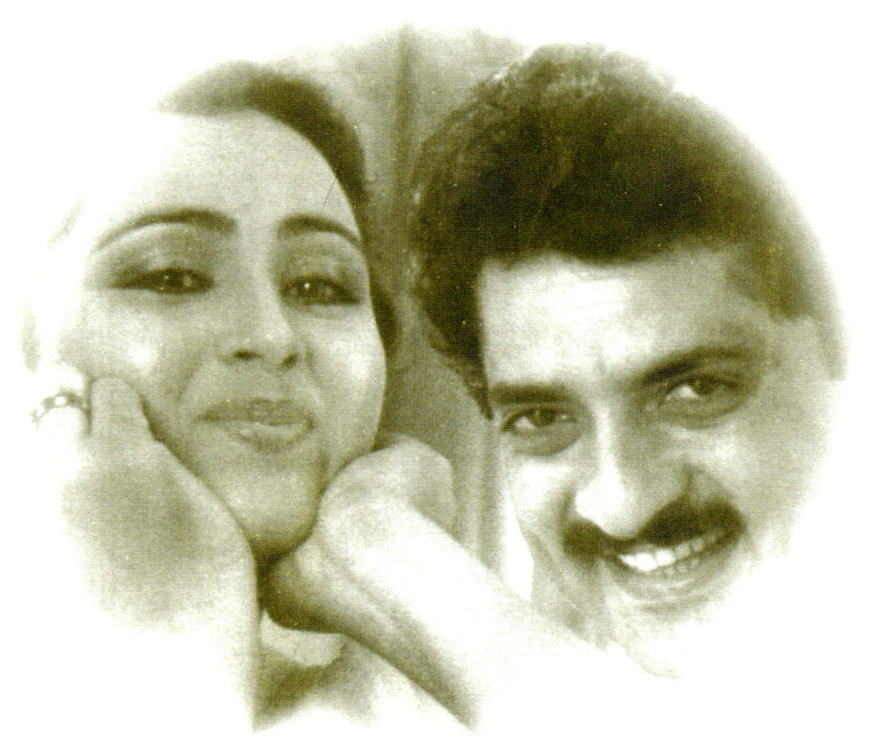

"It is so characteristic, that just when the mechanics of reproduction are so vastly improved, there are fewer and fewer people who know how the music should be played."

-Ludwig Wittgenstein (1889-1951),
Austrian philosopher.

Are You Ready to Have a Baby ?

Thinking ahead and planning well in advance is generally a sure recipe for a happy ending. This age-old wisdom applies equally well to parenthood. You can avoid several potential risks to the baby simply by being aware of them and acting to a plan. The chapter also discusses when a woman is most fertile in her life and how she can calculate the day of her egg release.

To be good parents, you must plan ahead. That is because your health and behaviour in pregnancy can affect your unborn baby. Certain illnesses, pills and medicines, smoking, risks at the work place... and other things can affect the baby's development or even cause abnormalities in a baby. The early months of pregnancy are especially important. Within the first 12 weeks of conception, the baby's organs are formed, including the brain, the nervous system and the heart. Yet during this vital time you may not even know that you are pregnant. Therefore, since no couple can know exactly when they will conceive, it makes sense to 'prepare' for pregnancy. Then you can be certain that from the moment of conception onwards you will be giving your baby the best possible chance of being healthy.

You should also know which are the best years for you to try and have a baby, and on which days of the monthly cycle you stand the best chance. Most couples succeed without trying too hard, but it is always better to know the basics of conceiving.

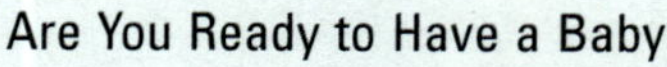

Mark Out Your Best Years

If you are a working woman, changing nappies may not be the first item on your plan. You may wish to excel in your career and then take a shot at the joys of motherhood. Sure, why not? Except that the doctors in the reproductive medicine field think it is not a good idea. A number of scientific studies on fertility affirm that a woman's best chance at motherhood lies in her early twenties. The first such investigation to probe into the relationship between fertility and a woman's age was carried out by Mathews Duncan many years ago. Checking on the fertility of women of different ages, he found maximum fertility between the ages of 19 and 25. The hard fact is, the female reproductive system ages faster than the other parts of the body—menopause at mid-life is the most striking sign—yet it is only a full stop at the end of the fertility chapter, decline sets in much earlier. Chances of fertility begin to dip by the age of 30, and become bleak in the forties.

A woman's eggs are affected by her age. The physiological aging of her ovaries lowers the fertility. Women over 30 who go for artificial insemination because their husbands have little or no sperms find it increasingly difficult to conceive, the egg being main limiting factor.

In contrast, if eggs of younger women are used, pregnancies are pretty much easy to come by. Even women well into menopause can nurture a pregnancy by using a younger woman's donor egg. It is the egg, rather than the uterus, which is the Achilles' heel of human reproduction. But surely, most women would not enjoy nestling another woman's egg.

So, it is best to go by Mother Nature's game plan. To enjoy motherhood, the age of 20 to 30 is the best. Beyond that, the amber light comes on. You could dash across it, or end up losing! The task becomes more and more difficult with each passing year. Between 30 and 35, a woman takes twice as long to conceive than she would 10 years earlier.

Deferring fertility is a gamble—you can win or lose. Your decision should be in this light.

Check Your Rubella Status

Catching rubella (German measles) in pregnancy is a sure shot invitation for disaster. The virus can severely damage the baby, especially if the mother catches the infection during the first three months of pregnancy. The baby's heart and nervous system can develop defects and the virus can also cause deafness and blindness in the baby. The mother may also suffer from miscarriage or stillbirth.

What to do

The best insurance against rubella is to get vaccinated. Check whether you were given the vaccine in your childhood. If not, ask your doctor for a vaccination now. This is one simple injection. You must also make sure that you do not get pregnant for the next three months after receiving the vaccination.

If you become pregnant without having received the shot against rubella and then come into contact with someone who has it, tell your doctor at once. A blood test will show whether or not you are naturally immune. If you are not, blood tests at fortnightly intervals will show whether you have been infected. If so, you have the option of ending your pregnancy.

When To Stop Contraceptives

If you are taking the contraceptive pill, it is probably best to stop about three months before you try to conceive. During these three months the best contraceptive to use is a condom or a cap, along with a spermicidal jelly. This gap between stopping the pill and starting a baby is useful because it allows your hormonal system to get back to normal. If your monthly cycle is back to normal before you conceive; you can be much more certain about when the baby will be due.

If you use a copper-T, then have it taken out at the end of a period. Then there is no need to wait before you try to conceive. The same is true for condoms, spermicidal jellies and caps.

Give Up Smoking

The dangers of smoking in pregnancy are many. It is known to harm the developing baby by retarding its growth and there is a risk that your baby will be born underweight. Babies of women who smoke are on an average 200 g lighter in weight. The nicotine that you inhale also makes its way into your baby. What is worse, the cigarette also passes in carbon monoxide into your bloodstream. Because of that, your blood oxygen level comes down and baby gets less oxygen. The risk of your baby being born premature is also high. You also run a bigger risk of complications when your baby is born.

What to do

Deciding to give up smoking, even for the sake of a baby, is not always simple. But if you mull over the gains, it is easy to be determined. Once you have made a decision to stop, you are half way there. Throw out all your cigarettes, lighters, matches and ashtrays. Get through without smoking for a day, then another, and then another. Eventually it begins to get easier and you begin to enjoy the benefits of not smoking. You may also find the following suggestions helpful:

- Find something to replace holding or playing with a cigarette. Doodle, knit, sew, play with a bunch of keys, twiddle your thumbs.
- Find other ways of relaxing. Do some deep breathing, take shower, go for a walk or a run, go swimming.
- Whenever you want to smoke, do something else. It does not matter what. Drink a glass of water, eat an apple, do one line of knitting, anything. Whatever you do, do not sit still and think about how much you want to smoke. If you cannot distract yourself this way, then at least divert your mind away.

Avoid Alcohol

Not just heavy drinking, but even moderate or light drinking, during pregnancy can affect the development of the baby adversely, especially during the early weeks. Whether you drink a lot or little, the alcohol that enters your bloodstream passes into your baby's bloodstream. And surely, that isn't a very pleasant thought!

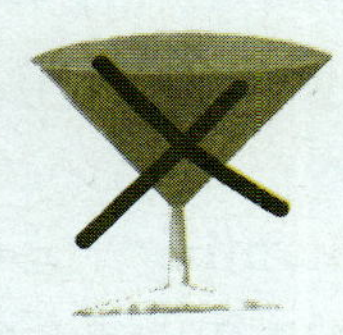

What to do

Cut out alcohol completely. Remember, from conception onwards, the less you drink, the better are your chances of a successful pregnancy and having a healthy baby. So, why take a risk? You can always find a non-alcoholic drink of your choice at social gatherings, and you do not necessarily have to state a reason for your changed preference.

Beware! Any Medicine Can Be Dangerous

A number of allopathic pills and medicines, including some that can be bought over the counter, can harm the developing baby. Even the most innocuous appearing ayurvedic, homeopathic and biochemical pills must be viewed with suspicion and are best left alone. The maximum harm is almost always done very early in pregnancy, when you still do not know that you are carrying.

What to do

If you are on any regular medication because of a chronic ailment, do not neglect to mention this fact to your doctor before you try to conceive. Conditions like epilepsy and diabetes require extra care during pregnancy to avoid any harm to the baby.

Ideally, healthy women should avoid all drugs unless they are prescribed by a qualified doctor. You must become particularly careful once you feel you may be with a baby.

Risks At the Work Place

It is possible that the work you do, especially certain sectors such as a nuclear reactor, chemical factory, noisy high-vibration machines, operating room environment, radiology or radiation treatment department could pose a threat to your baby's health. You could be at risk if you are exposed to radiation, work with certain chemicals, like mercury, benzene or lead, or the work you do is particularly tiring or stressful.

What to do

You must avoid taking any risk after conception. If you think you could be at risk, check with an authentic source without the slightest delay. Talk to your employer, union representative or personnel department. If there is a definite risk in what you do, you must ask to be moved to a job that is safe. For instance, typically, in a radiology department, the technician or the doctor is taken off duties where she may be exposed to radiation risk and put on work in an ultrasound

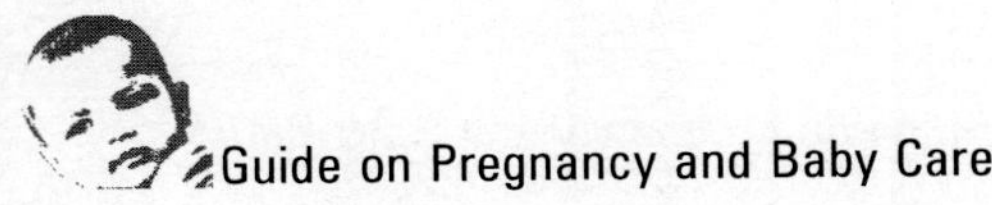

or reporting room. If such a change is not possible, you should decide upon a change of job.

Risks of An Inherited Abnormality

Just as characteristics like physical features such as shape of the nose and eyes are passed on in families through the genes, in the same way certain abnormalities can be genetically inherited. If either you or your partner suffers from a condition such as muscular dystrophy, Huntington's chorea, sickle cell disease or haemophilia, then you must know what sort of a risk you would be taking by having a baby.

The risk varies with the nature of defect and also, whether one or both parents carry the defect. Some defects are due to defects of a single gene. They are inherited in a simple fashion and the risk of their recurring in the family can be accurately predicted. The so-called autosomal dominant defects have a one in two chance of being carried forward if the defect is present in one parent. A number of defects fall under this category. They include haemoglobin defects, red blood cell defect (hereditary spherocytosis), liver defect (Gilbert's syndrome), brain and nervous system disorder (Hutington's chorea), muscular dystrophy, pathological fragility of bones (osteogenesis imperfecta), polycystic disease of kidneys, polyps in the large bowel, and others. In contrast to these dominant defects, the recessive traits are transmitted much less commonly and often do not lead to a disease unless two persons carrying the same defect marry and have children. In this eventuality, there is a one in four chance at conception that the baby will be born with the defect. Such defects include albinism, cystic fibrosis, Fanconi syndrome, phenylketonuria, thalassaemia, Wilson's disease,

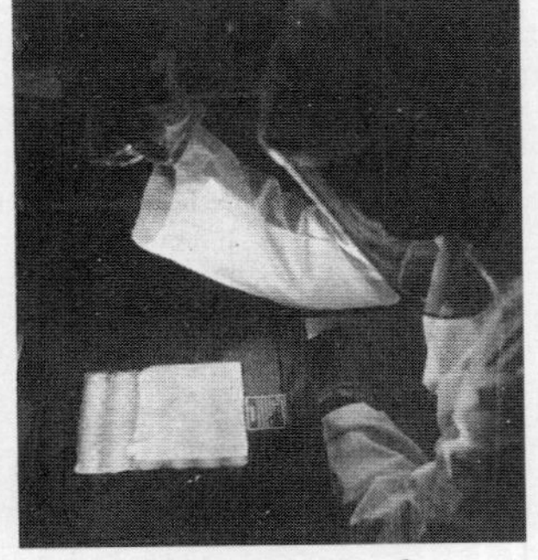

A geneticist at work

and a host of others. A third category of defects is one that is inherited as sex-linked. This category has two sub categories: one that is dominant and is found to affect both males and females, while the other in which females are healthy carriers and transmit the disease to their male children, the classical example being that of haemophilia, a disorder marked by defect in normal blood clotting mechanism of the body.

The list of single gene defects is very large and if there is a family history of any such defect the best course is to discuss with your doctor about the risk of any such abnormality passing on to a foetus.

Estimated risk for some common disorders

Disorder	How Common	Male: Female Ratio	Normal parents having a second affected child	Affected parent having an affected child	Affected parent having a second affected child
Absence of head	2 per1000	1:2	5%	—	—
Cleft palate	4 per 10,000	2:3	2%	7%	15%
Cleft lip ± cleft palate	1 per1000	3:2	4%	4%	10%
Club foot	1 per1000	2:1	3%	3%	10%
Heart defects	1 per 200	—	1-4%	1-4%	—
Dislocation of hip	7 per10,000	1:6	4%	4%	10%
Epilepsy	1 per 200	1:1	5%	5%	10%
Maniac illness	1 per 250	2:3	—	10-15%	—
Mental retardation	1 per 200	1:1	3-5%	—	—
Deafness	1 per1000	1:1	10%	8%	—
Absence of both kidneys	1 per10,000	3:1	3-7%	—	—
Obstruction at the stomach outlet (Pyloric stenosis)	3 per1000	5:1	2-10%	4-17%	13-38%
Schizophrenia	1-2 per 100	1:1	—	16%	—
Spinal bone defect	3 per1000	2:3	5%	3%	—

A genetic counsellor can tell you more clearly about the sort of risk you would be taking.

The transmissibility of many common disorders is even more complex. They are inherited on a multifactorial basis and many genes plus the effects of environment are thought to play an important part in their occurrence. The empiric risk score for some such disorders is presented here (see table).

Even if there is a high risk of having a child with a serious genetic disorder, couples can always exercise their option of asking for an antenatal diagnosis through amniocentesis around the 16th week of pregnancy and if the foetus is affected of aborting it. A couple can also use donor egg or sperms depending on the defect and its seriousness.

When Are You Most Likely To Conceive?

A woman is most likely to conceive just after the time she ovulates. The egg lives for about 24 hours after it is released from the ovary. If you are going to conceive, the egg has to be fertilised within these 24 hours. Again the sperm lives only for 48 to 72 hours. So, the best time to conceive is around the date that you are likely to have the ovulation. This allows the sperm to travel up into the fallopian tubes and meet the egg.

How to find out when you ovulate

The calendar method

1 If your monthly cycle is fairly regular, you are probably used to working out when your next period is due. You can work out the ovulation time the same way. First, you have to know the pattern of your monthly cycle. Keep a record of your periods. Each month, mark the first day of your bleeding in your diary or calendar. Do this

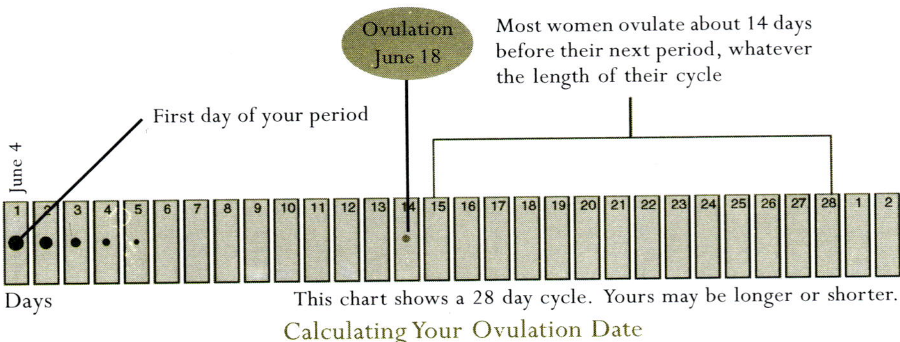

Calculating Your Ovulation Date

for a number of months.

2 You can now work out the length of your monthly cycle by counting the days, from the first day of one period up to the first day of the next. If you have a regular cycle, the number of days between your periods will be about the same each month. But if the number varies a lot, you obviously have an irregular cycle and you will need to use other methods such as temperature or mucus methods to find out when you ovulate.

3 The length of menstrual cycle varies in most women. Still, most women ovulate about 14 days before their next period. So using what you know to be the usual length of your monthly cycle, work out the first day of your next period. Now count back 14 days and you have the time when you are likely to ovulate

The temperature method

Just after you ovulate, your temperature first drops a little and then goes up. So keeping a record of your temperature is another way of finding out when you ovulate. If you are having difficulty conceiving, your doctor may advise you to keep a temperature chart because it can show not only when you are ovulating but whether or not you are ovulating at all.

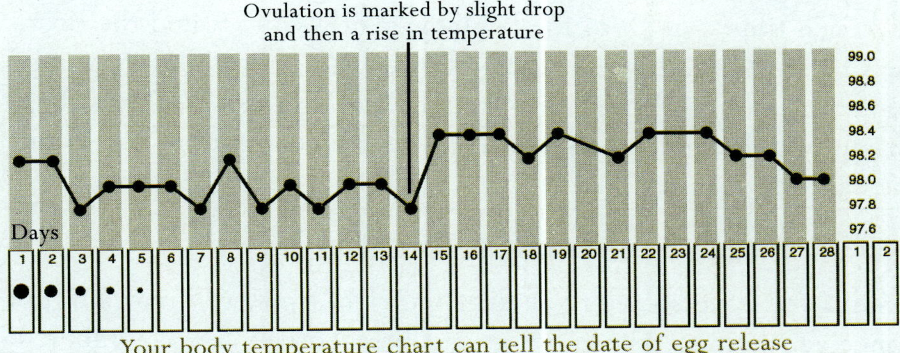

Your body temperature chart can tell the date of egg release

1. Starting on the first day of a period take your temperature first thing in the morning. Use a special 'fertility' thermometer which you can buy from a chemist. Keep the thermometer in your mouth for a good two minutes.
2. Keep an everyday record of your temperature in the form of a chart.
3. On the first day of your next period, start a new chart.
4. You will observe that about 14 days before your period commenced, your temperature would record a slight drop and then go up.
5. When your temperature rises, you have already ovulated. Since an egg can live in the fallopian tube for about 24 hours you can still conceive if you have an intercourse.

The mucus method

Just before you ovulate, the mucus around the cervix becomes thinner so that it is easier for sperm to travel through it. There is also more mucus produced. Some women notice this around the middle of their monthly cycle when there is much more wetness around the vagina. Others get a clear, jelly-like discharge. These are both signs that ovulation is about to happen.

Each time you go to the lavatory, gently wipe round the opening of the vagina with your fingers or a tissue. On the days around ovulation, you will find more mucus and wetness. At first these changes can be difficult to recognise, but if you are more observant, they are easy to pick.

How Long Does It Usually Take To Conceive?

Even if you have an intercourse at the right time, you may still not conceive. Women who have used contraceptives for a number of years often think that as soon as they stop using it, they will become pregnant. But in a real life situation, it does not work like that. It is quite normal for a woman to take many months to conceive. Only if, you do not conceive after trying for one full year should you think of asking for a doctor's advice. Go to your doctor and explain your worry.

A failure to conceive can be due to physical causes such as the man producing too few sperms or the sperm conducting apparatus being blocked, the woman failing to ovulate or the fallopian tubes being blocked, or the marriage not being consummated. Many of these problems can be treated. Sometimes psychological difficulties also count. Failing to conceive can also be the result of being over-anxious, tired or tense. Whatever may be the cause, take your doctor's advice. Professional insight can soon put you on the road to parenthood.

Can You Choose Your Baby's Sex?

This question has intrigued common men and professionals for a long while. The basis of their deduction is not known, but flipping through some of the ancient medical texts, many interesting beliefs come to light. There are dates and days to go by, postures to adopt and food items to be eaten.

If only the rules had been that simple! Much as we have progressed in reproductive medicine, creating babies in test tubes and petri-dishes, siphoning off eggs from donors, shopping for wombs on rent, there are mysteries that continue to riddle the human mind regarding determination of the sex of a baby in the mother's womb.

Nobody knows the conditions which favour the 'X' sperm or the 'Y' sperm to fertilise the egg and begin new life. Of the masterly game-plan, the key to which only Mother Nature knows, science has only been able to figure that when an 'X' sperm mates with the egg, a girl baby is born and if a 'Y' sperm fertilises the egg, the baby will be a boy. The statistical probabilities are even. Sperms of either type can play their part and that is a sheer chance. Neither the man nor the woman can be the deciding factor. That truly is one way the Mother Nature maintains the balance.

It is astonishing that many neem-hakims still publicly sell magic pills and potions to enable you to choose your baby's sex. Buses, trains and walls of buildings are defaced by alluring advertisements inviting you to sample their wares. Many couples get enticed into visiting such quacks. They perhaps do not realise that once this natural selection has occurred no pill howsoever magical it may be can alter the sex of the baby. You may argue against this by saying that such potions do work. Believe us, if they do, it is simply because Nature allows them an even chance to succeed. All quacks owe their reputation to sheer chance. Their prey are the gullible and even if they were to give sugar pills, the laws of Nature would have ensured the success of the quacks five times out of ten.

The innumerable old wives' tales about foretelling the baby's gender on the basis of would-be mother's style of walking, her food preferences, her dreams and many such plausible body signals also have no scientific sanction.

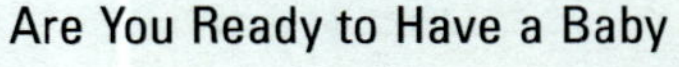

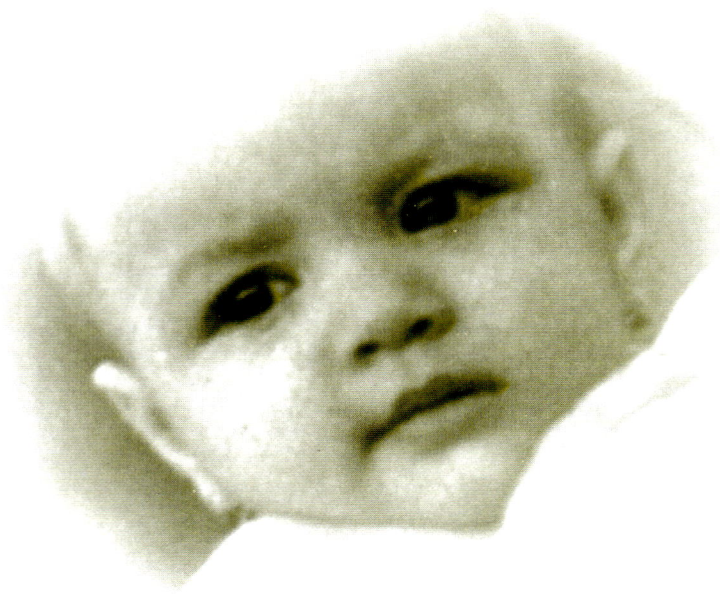

*"Luckless is the country in
which the symbols of procreation are
the objects of shame,
while the agents of destruction are honoured!
And yet you call that member your pudendum,
or shameful part, as if there were anything
more glorious than creating life,
or anything more atrocious
than taking it away."*

-Cyrano de Bergerac (1619-55), French author, playwright.
A "Lunarian," in The Other World: States and Empires of the Moon.

What Makes Babies ?

Much has changed since Mother Nature created man. Armed with test tubes, petri dishes and microscopes, modern man's sapience today allows him to set up a brave new world. The much-talked technique of cloning has facilitated the birth of the sheep Dolly from a single breast tissue cell taken from a 'sister', or shall we say, 'mother' sheep. And more recently, mouse Fibro, now perhaps no less known than Mickey, has been born - all from a single cell taken from his father's tail! Nature's game plan has truly been turned upside down, but the rules for human reproduction have largely not changed. The beginning of a new human life is still generally sparked in bedrooms rather than science labs. A man and a woman meet in sexual union for the seeds of life, one from the mother and the other from the father, to fuse and begin the 40-week journey of developing into a baby.

Human beings are equipped with a wonderful reproductive system. That has enabled mankind to survive on this planet for millions of years. Our bodies begin to produce the seeds of life from puberty. Mature girls produce eggs or ova till their forties, while men produce sperms all their life. It just needs a sperm to penetrate the egg and spark a new life. Our complex machinery works itself into readiness for a large part of our lives, unmindful of the waste! With totally different roles to play, the sexual machineries of man and woman are, however, altogether different. Let us take a brief look at their design and the way they function.

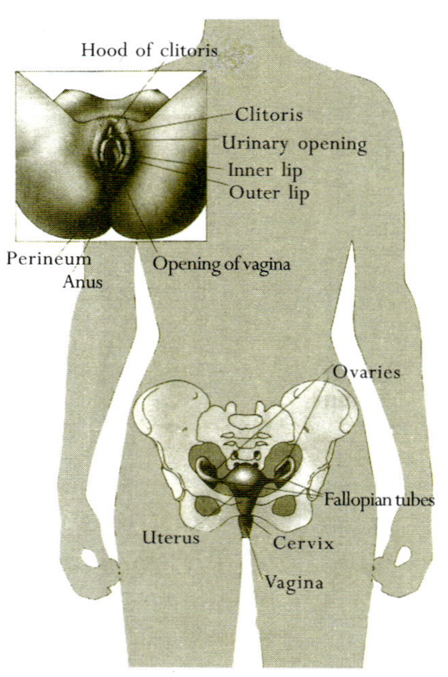

Female Sexual System

External sex organs

Vulva

Vulva is the name given to the external sex organs of the female. It has several parts, the most obvious being the labia majora (large lips).

Labia majora

When a woman is standing it appears as a narrow slit which comes together in the midline. The large lips are composed mainly of fat and small glands that lubricate the vaginal canal.

Clitoris

Mons pubis

The mons pubis is a pad of fat that lies over the pubic bone. Hair appears in this area at puberty.

Labia minora

Just under labia majora are two smaller, more sensitive folds called the labia minora (small lips). Labia minora meet in front and upper part of the clitoris.

Clitoris

This is an extremely sensitive erectile organ. It is analogous to the male penis in many ways, and its stimulation during an intercourse is crucial to enjoyment of sex and attainment of orgasm.

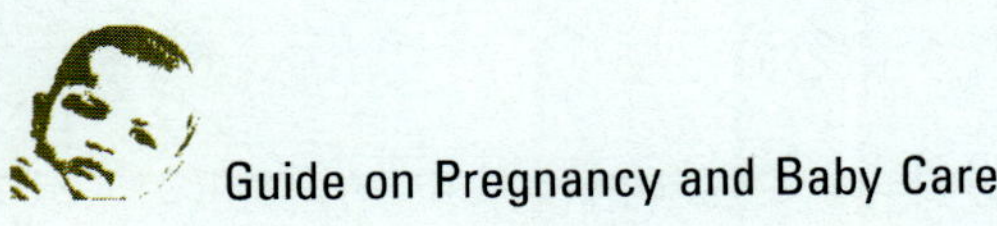

Urethral Orifice

A little below clitoris is a small opening through which urine flows. This is the urethral orifice.

Vaginal Orifice

Immediately below the urethral opening is the opening to the vaginal canal called the vaginal orifice.

Bartholin's Glands

Bartholin's glands are two small bean-shaped glands, one on either side of the vaginal opening. These glands normally secrete a lubricating fluid which facilitates the act of intercourse.

Vagina

Vagina is located above the rectum and below the urethra. It is about three to four inches deep, and extends upwards and inwards at an angle to end at the cervix (the opening to the uterus). Being very elastic, it is capable of considerable expansion. It receives the male organ during an intercourse and is the first receptacle to receive the sperms.

The vagina has a natural lubrication system. It remains moist with the moistness varying throughout the menstrual cycle and when a woman is sexually aroused.

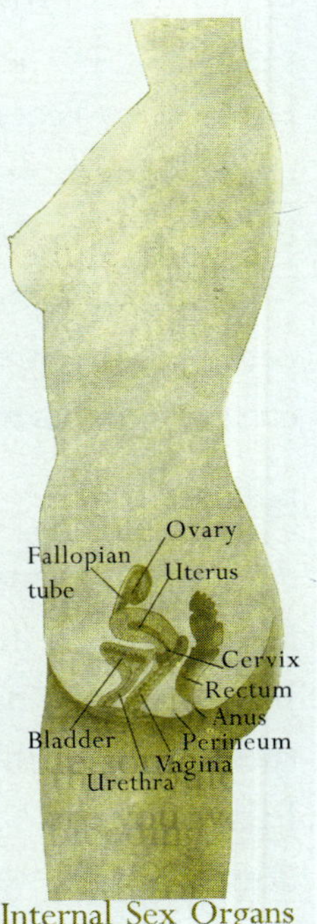

Internal Sex Organs

Internal Sex Organs

Cervix

The vaginal canal opens at its upper end into the cervix or the narrow outer end of the uterus. The

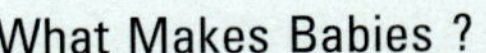

glands in the cervix produce mucus which changes in nature with the phase of menstrual cycle. The female sex hormones, oestrogen and progesterone, guide this change. During the fertile period, the mucus allows easy entry to the sperms.

Uterus (Womb)

The uterus (womb) is a pear-shaped, hollow, muscular organ approximately three inches long, two inches wide, and one inch thick. It has a cavity inside which can undergo remarkable changes in size. It nests and nurtures the developing baby.

The uterus sits in the pelvis in the midline and tilts forward. It is lined with a special tissue called the endometrium. The thickness of this varies from day to day, according to the day of the menstrual cycle. The hormones formed by the ovaries control this change. They fatten it to receive the fertilised egg. If the egg is not fertilised, the uterus sheds its tissue resulting in menstruation. This cyclical bleeding lasts three to seven days in a month till a woman is fertile.

The main portion of the uterus is called the body and the uppermost part is referred to as the fundus. At the upper corner of the uterus on each side, a narrow canal leads out and joins the fallopian tube.

Fallopian Tubes

About four inches in length, each of the two Fallopian tubes, on their far end, open in close approximation with ovaries of corresponding side. They are not attached to the ovaries but surround and envelop them. The ovum (egg) on its release from the ovary is swept into the Fallopian tube by natural suction and continues its movement downwards toward the uterus. The hair-like cilia present in the walls of the Fallopian tube assist the ovum in its journey. The mating of ovum with sperm, a process called fertilisation, normally occurs in the Fallopian tube. If the Fallopian tubes are blocked, pregnancy remains an unfulfilled dream without proper medical help.

Ovaries

The ovaries are located on either side of the uterus and contain between 200,000 and 400,000 ova (eggs) at the time of birth. They also produce the hormones oestrogen and progesterone.

Each ovary is a whitish-grey organ about the size and shape of an almond. It is packed with thousands of microscopic partially developed eggs which have been present since birth. After a woman attains sexual maturity, each month, one or more eggs mature and get released from the ovary. This process is called ovulation. It occurs about once in every four weeks and is part of the preparation for fertilisation and pregnancy. When a woman is pregnant, this process takes a rest. It resumes its regular pattern only a few months after the birth of the baby. In a normal reproductive life span, a woman releases only about 450 eggs from her ovaries. The remaining eggs are simply lost over time.

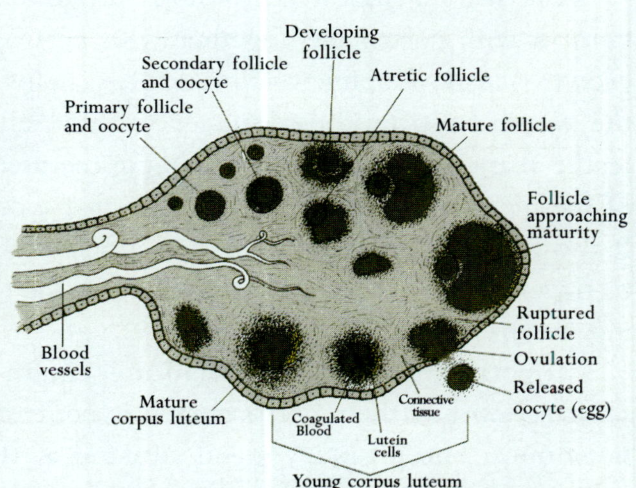

A woman's ovary houses eggs in different stages of development

Female Sex Hormones And What They Do

The two basic sex hormones in a woman are oestrogen and progesterone. Both are produced in the ovaries and to a smaller extent in the adrenals. It is due to the secretion of these hormones that a girl finds her way to sexual maturity in her teen years. They also play a key role in her menstrual cycle.

Oestrogen serves many useful functions. When a girl reaches puberty it facilitates the growth and development of external sex organs–the breasts, uterus, Fallopian tubes and the ovaries. The shapely contours of her body with narrow shoulders and broad hips are also attributed to this hormone. It also aids in the maturation of her bones. Once a girl attains maturity, oestrogen keeps her uterus and other sex organs in good health. It rebuilds the inner lining of the uterus every month following its shedding at the time of menstruation and thus prepares the ground for a fertilised egg to set in.

The second master hormone is progesterone which works in tandem with oestrogen. Together with oestrogen it stimulates the growth and development of breasts and helps the muscle fibres of the womb to grow during puberty. Later, all through a woman's fertile years it helps fatten the lining of the uterus in the second half of the menstrual cycle in anticipation that a conception may occur. It also increases the motility of the Fallopian tubes to assist the ovum to travel towards the uterus and enhances the growth of uterus during pregnancy.

Together, these two hormones maintain the organs of procreation but their performance is controlled by the pituitary hormones. The pituitary gland situated at the base of the brain activates the ovaries for the onset of the menstrual cycle.

The Menstrual Cycle

During her active reproductive years, beginning at puberty, when she is 10 to 16 years of age till she reaches menopause, at the age of 45 to 50, a woman goes through a very special cycle. This cycle or rhythm is the show of her fertility and carries a very special meaning for her.

In this cycle, once in every 28 days or so (it varies a little in every woman), the lining of the uterus is gradually shed. This process which extends anywhere from two to seven days is termed the menstrual period. The outset of the cycle is marked by blood discharge. It has many colloquial names and whenever a woman uses quaint names it is not difficult to understand what she is referring to.

The mechanisms that regulate the build up and shedding of the uterine lining are controlled by changes in body's hormone levels. The two pituitary hormones, the follicle stimulating hormone (FSH) and the luteinising hormone govern this cycle. The pituitary gland releases them into the bloodstream and they race away to the ovaries. The ovaries hold the eggs in their inactive form called follicles. During each cycle, FSH and LH stimulate one or more of these follicles to ripen and be released from the ovary for a

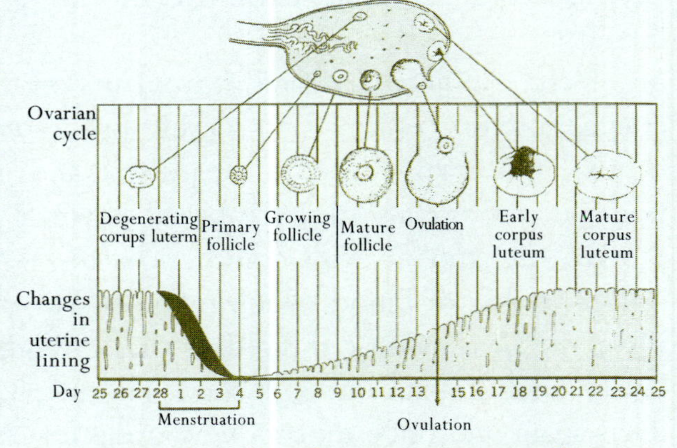

Menstrual Cycle : Changes in Ovaries and Uterus

possible fertilisation. The follicles are no laggards; they also produce the hormones oestrogen and progesterone. Oestrogen works the hardest during the first half of the cycle as the egg is undergoing maturation, while progesterone is the dominant hormone after the egg is released.

It is oestrogen which helps the uterine lining to gradually rebuild in two weeks, following menstruation. The inner mucous layer of glands of the endometrium (uterine lining), begins to grow long and the lining thickens with an increase in the number of blood vessels as well as the production of a mesh of fibres that interconnect throughout the lining. By about day 14, or mid cycle, the lining of the uterus thickens to about three times as compared to the beginning of the cycle. Its blood supply also increases considerably.

Around day 14, ovulation occurs; the egg is released from the ovary at the signal of the luteinising hormone. This egg is picked up by the Fallopian tube and it continues on its onward journey towards the uterus. The follicle from which the egg is released is stimulated by the luteinising hormone. It changes into a yellow body called the corpus luteum. It is the corpus luteum that secretes progesterone. Progesterone stimulates the uterine lining to grow further and fatten.

If the egg gets fertilised, it implants on the uterine wall and the corpus luteum continues to secrete progesterone. If no fertilisation occurs, the corpus luteum dies down and progesterone dips. The lining of the uterus starts to break down leading to menstruation. Slowly, the uterine wall commences to crumble. At first there is only a trickle of blood which finds its way out through the vagina. Over the next two or three days the flow increases until finally the entire endometrial lining is shed. The uterine wall begins to build itself again and once more a new cycle begins.

Male Sexual System

In men, the reproductive system is equally elaborate. It includes the testes, a duct system, some accessory glands, and the penis. The testes are the organs that produce sperms. The duct system, which includes the epididymis and the vas deferens, transports the sperms. The accessory glands, mainly the seminal vesicles and the prostate gland, provide fluids that lubricate the duct system and nourish the sperm. The penis, a cylindrical organ located between the legs releases sperms at the height of sexual excitement.

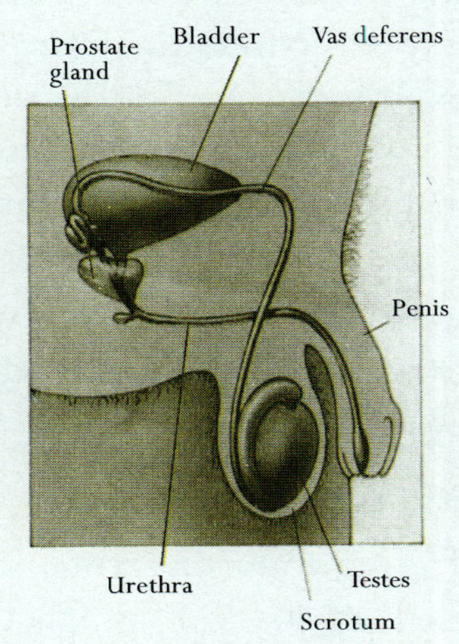

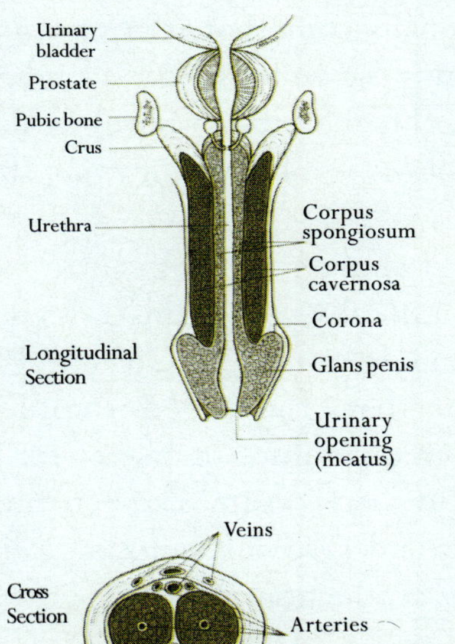

Structure of Penis

Penis

The penis is made of spongy tissues that contain small blood vessels and nerves. It has three columns of erectile tissue: the two corpora cavernosa placed side by side, and the corpus spongiosum behind them. The end of the corpus spongiosum is enlarged to form the conical tip (glans penis). The glans is smooth and contains many nerve endings making it extremely sensitive.

At the very tip of the glans is the urethral opening through which urine

and semen leave the body. A loose fold of skin called the prepuce or foreskin covers the glans. It is like a hood and can be rolled back to expose the head of the penis.

When a man is sexually stimulated the arterial blood vessels in the penis expand causing more blood to flow into it. At the same time, reflex contraction of muscle fibres compresses the penile veins that drain away the blood. As a result, blood cannot exit. This expands the spongy tissues within the penis making it grow large and become rigid.

Scrotum

The scrotum or scrotal sac is a thin-walled, soft, muscular pouch. Each of its two compartments holds the testes or testicles. The scrotum automatically responds to changes in temperature. If the outside temperature rises and conditions become hot, the scrotum becomes very loose and soft. This allows the testes to hang farther from the body. In contrast, if it gets cold, the muscle fibres in the scrotum cause the entire sac to contract or wrinkle up, drawing the testes closer to the body.

The scrotum thus acts as a natural climate control centre for the testes. The temperature in the scrotum always remains a degree or two lower than the usual body temperature of 37°C (98.6°F). The testes produce sperms, and for that, they need a cooler temperature. If the testes are at body temperature or higher for a prolonged period, infertility or sterility can result. The scrotum continually monitors the environment and responds automatically in a way that is best for healthy sperm production.

Testes

The testes are the two small balls that hang in the scrotum below the penis. Oval in shape, each testis measures about 1½ inch long,

1 inch wide and 1¼ inch across and weighs about an ounce each. In most men, the left testis is a bit heavier and larger and hangs a little lower than the right. The reason why this should be so is not known, but it may be to stop the testicles from striking each other as the man walks.

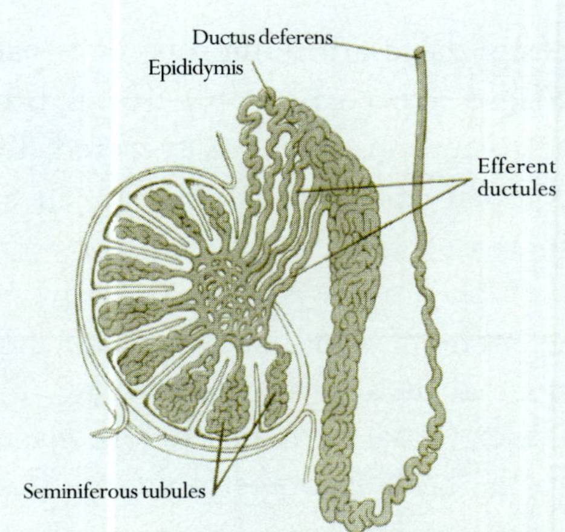

Sperm manufacturing units in the testis and the duct system that transports the sperms

The testes have two functions: to produce sperms from puberty until death, and to produce male sex hormones called androgens, of which testosterone is the most important. A healthy adult male normally produces about 200 million sperms per day, although there is a decline with age.

Sperms are produced in the testis in special structures called seminiferous tubules. These tubes are in the centre of the testis and connected with a series of passageways that convey the sperms through the male reproductive tract and ultimately out of the penis if required.

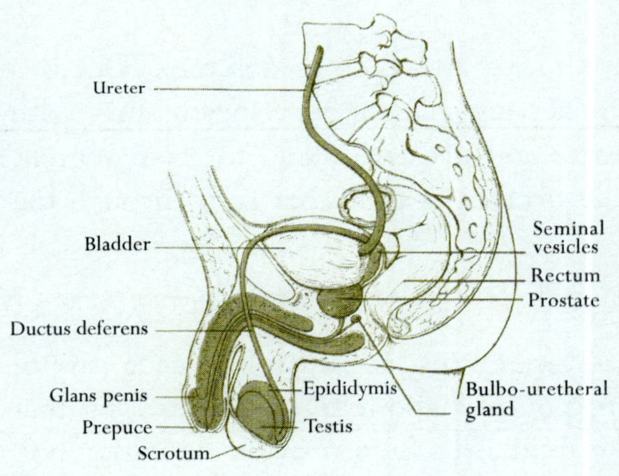

Male Sexual System

Near the seminiferous tubules in each

testis there are numerous cells called interstitial or Leydig's cells. These are responsible for producing the male sex hormone, testosterone, which is secreted directly into nearby blood vessels. Majority of physical changes in a boy, at puberty are due to the increased amount of testosterone flowing through his body.

The testes also go through a series of changes during sexual excitement. For one, their size increases to one-and-a-half times of normal because of the increase in blood flow. And two, they draw closer to the body just before ejaculation. The testes also draw close to the body in times of intense fear and anger.

Epididymis

On the upper posterior portion of each testis, there is a slight ridge. This is the epididymis. It is a tightly coiled tube which adheres to the surface of the testis and acts as a maturation and storage chamber for the newly developed sperms. Sperms stay in the epididymes until they break down and are absorbed by the surrounding tissue or until they are ejaculated.

Vas deferens

From the epididymis sperms move into the vas deferens. This is a long tube about 16 to 18 inches long. In the vas, sperms mix with fluids from the seminal vesicle and prostate gland to form semen. The vas deferens leads to the urethra, a tube that runs through the penis.

Seminal vesicles

The two seminal vesicles are located just above and on each side of the prostate gland. They are pouches about three inches long that secrete fructose, a sugar-like fluid. This fluid provides nutrition and energy to the sperms, enabling them to move more effectively.

Prostate gland

The prostate gland is situated below the neck of the bladder, encircling the urethra. It produces a thin, milky, alkaline fluid that is secreted into the urethra at the time of emission of semen, providing an added medium for the life and motility of sperm.

The prostatic fluid makes 95 percent of the semen, while fluid from the seminal vesicles contributes about four percent; and the remaining one percent alone is made up of sperms.

Expulsion of Semen

The process of expulsion of the semen through the male urethra is called ejaculation. This process takes place at the height of sexual excitement. A wave of contraction sweeps over the muscles around the male reproductive organs forcing a sudden forceful emission of semen through the penile urethra. The amount of semen ejaculated at any one time varies between two to six millilitres and each millilitre contains about 60 to 120 million sperms.

Conception

For pregnancy to begin, a sperm must fertilise an egg. Fertilisation also called conception, occurs by means of copulation or sexual intercourse, wherein a male inserts an erect penis into the female vagina. When the male ejaculates, millions of sperms get deposited in the vagina.

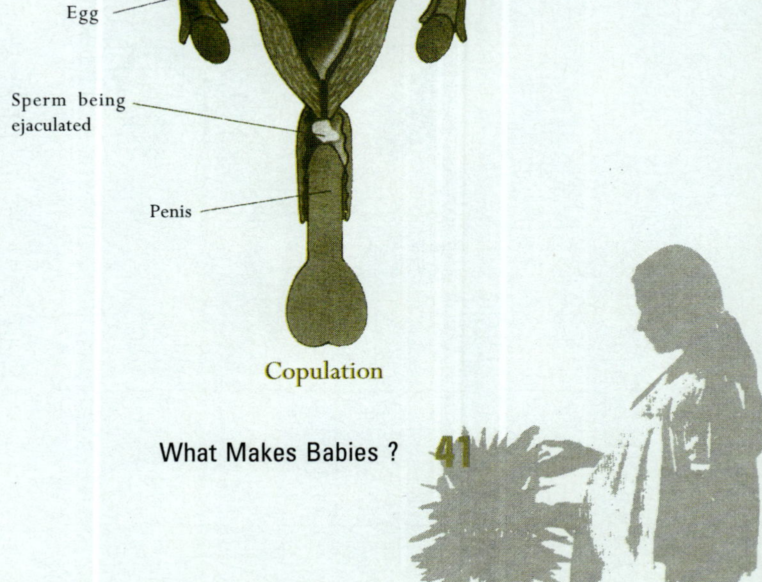

Copulation

The same can be replicated by artificial means without a sexual intercourse. In a process known as artificial insemination, semen is collected beforehand from a man and injected into the vagina. In another technique, called in vitro fertilisation (IVF, more popularly known as the test tube baby technique), sperms are used to fertilise eggs in a laboratory dish. A fertilised egg is then inserted into the woman's uterus.

In the normal process of conception following ejaculation, the sperms swim across very quickly through the vagina into the uterus and into the fallopian tubes. Many die on the way, but no less than a few thousand reach the tubes. Some are quick and take as little as five minutes to reach the spot, while others are slow and take a few hours. In any case, their useful life is simply between 48 to 72 hours. If an egg comes through during this period, they try their best to fertilise it. The surface of a newly released egg is covered with a jellylike layer of cells called the zona pellucida. A second layer, called the cumulus oophorus, surrounds the zona pellucida. A sperm must pass through both layers to fertilise the egg. The acrosome or the tip of the sperm releases special enzymes that scatter the cells of both layers. Although several sperm may swamp the zona pellucida, usually it is only one which makes the final grade mating with the egg. As the first sperm enters, the egg draws close its doors. It releases substances that prevent other sperms from entering.

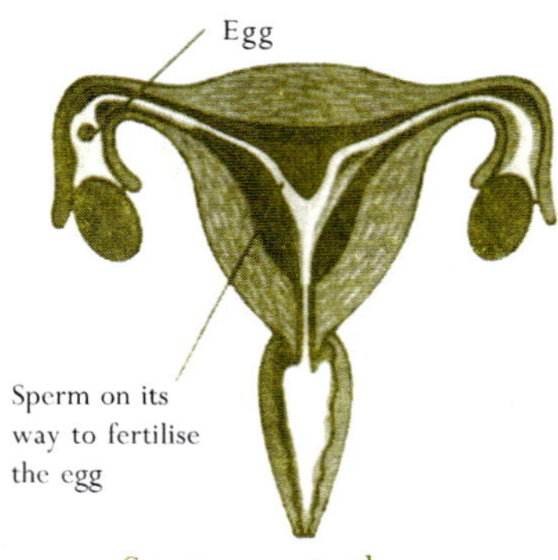

Sperm meets the egg

The union mostly occurs in the outer portion of one of the fallopian tubes. The chromosomes of the sperm unite with the

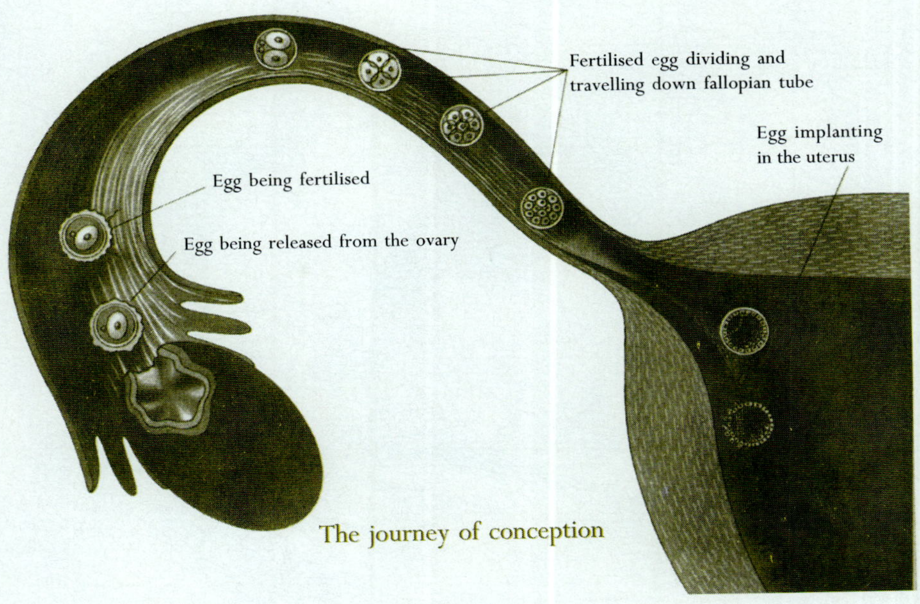

The journey of conception

chromosomes of the egg, making a total number of 46 chromosomes. The fertilised egg, now called a zygote, travels to the uterus, which waits in all readiness. During its journey, which takes three to five days, it quickly subdivides, then re-divides and continues to divide. The number of cells double on each occasion. By the time it reaches the uterus it has developed into a mass of cells. The embryo develops from the central cells, while the peripheral cells shape into the placenta. For details pertaining to this process of development of the embryo into a full grown baby turn to page 52.

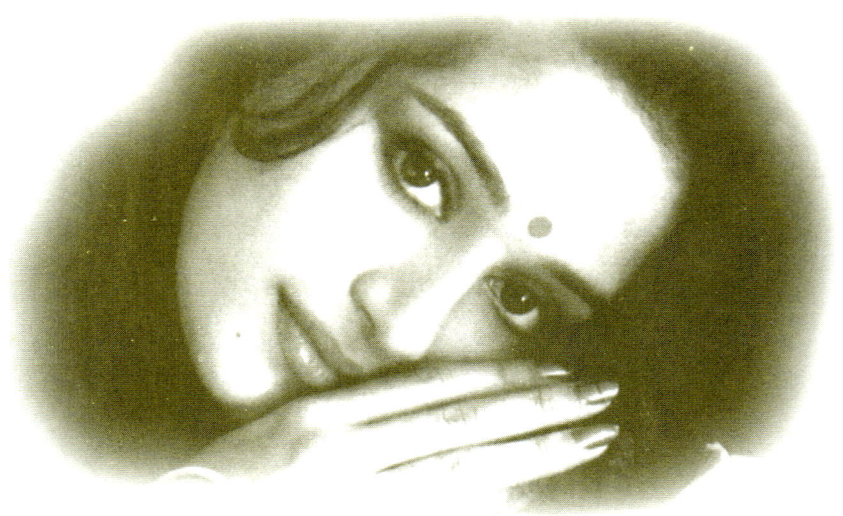

What sweet dreams
Quietly fill her being
Songs of great rejoice
Revel her soul!
"Spread out I would
A bed of nectar for him
Rocking the craddle
I would caress him."

-Jaishankar Prasad (1890-1937),
Kamayani.

Knowing that You Are Pregnant

Because pregnancy changes a woman's normal hormone patterns, one of the first signs of pregnancy is a missed menstrual period. But many women know intuitively that they are with a child. For others, there are many other symptoms as well. A do-it-yourself pregnancy test done soon after you miss the period can settle the issue 99 times out of 100 and a pelvic ultrasound, at six weeks, can remove all doubts.

So, you think you are pregnant!

You have just missed your period and are overdue.

There is that unpleasant feeling of nausea and you do not feel very well.

You visit the toilet more often—sometimes even during the night.

There is an increased vaginal discharge, without any soreness or irritation.

You have suddenly becoming finicky towards smells.

You find your breasts are changing. They have got bigger and feel tender and tingle. The veins have started to show up and the nipples have become darker and stand out.

You feel constipated.

There are cravings for unusual substances such as tamarind, clay or ice.

Yes, you are likely to be right! It does appear that you are on your way to becoming a mother. The developing zygote (fertilised egg) in the uterus is generating a progressive wave of structural and functional changes in you. You already have begun to show the first signs. Now, you must be careful. These first few months are very critical for your baby. During this period, the baby's brain, arms, legs, and internal organs are formed. Do not take any medication, avoid all X-rays and stop smoking and consuming alcohol. It is one of those precious times when you would blossom to nurture and give birth to a new life. Enjoy the occasion as your body experiences a number of firsts.

The First Symptoms

The first symptoms are just as you described—stoppage of menses, morning sickness, frequent passage of urine, swelling of the breasts, enlargement of the belly and 'quickening'. But you must know that not one of these symptoms occurring singly nor all of them occurring together can be looked upon as a conclusive evidence of pregnancy. They need a confirmation by doing special tests. But let us go over these symptoms first.

Stoppage of Menses

The cessation of menses or amenorrhoea is the first symptom that brings to attention the possibility of pregnancy. Unusually, however, regular menstruation may continue for the first two or three months in a few pregnant women. Occasionally, this symptom of amenorrhoea may also occur without pregnancy. Girls in their late teens or early twenties may experience amenorrhoea as a result of change in occupation or surroundings. Anxiety and stress may also delay the menstrual flow. It is best not to panic, unless there is reason to, in which case it is best to get a thorough check-up.

This symptom also affords the best means of estimating the duration of pregnancy. It is usual to reckon the beginning of pregnancy from the first day of the last regular menstrual period. This method is sometimes fallacious, for pregnancy may occur during an interval of amenorrhoea due to some other reason such as suckling. It takes no account of the fact that the date of fruitful sexual intercourse does not quite correspond with the date of last menstrual period, yet it is the best available method.

Morning Sickness

This symptom is by no means invariable in pregnancy. A great majority of first-time mothers suffer from it but in subsequent pregnancies it is frequently absent. It usually appears at the beginning of the second month, soon after the first suppressed period and it varies in severity. Some pregnant women are seized with nausea, ending in vomiting immediately on rising in the morning or after their first meal. There is no further discomfort or loss of appetite during the rest of the day. Others are subject to nausea, without vomiting, which may last for several hours and is very bothersome. It usually lasts for only a few weeks and rarely for more than three months.

Frequency of Urination

The woman usually notices a marked desire to pass urine, though very scantily. There is usually no burning sensation or fever that occurs in bladder and urinary tract infections. It is simply the physiological changes occurring in the pelvic area which cause irritability of the bladder. This symptom is common during the second and third months of pregnancy, and is caused by the pressure of the growing uterus and in part by congestion of the inner lining layer of the bladder. After the third month, when the uterus rises above the pelvic brim and becomes more erect the pressure is removed and this symptom disappears.

Changes in the Breasts

During the first pregnancy breasts undergo a series of changes, many of which persist into later life. The whole gland increases in size and undergoes a true enlargement. This enlargement is first recognisable in the outer lobules of the gland which become tense, nodular, and slightly tender to the touch. This process begins about the end of the second month and becomes more pronounced as the pregnancy advances. When the enlargement of the lobules is well marked, a little clear pale-yellow secretion can usually be seen by gently compressing the periphery of the gland and squeezing it towards the nipple. The secretion varies in texture during pregnancy. When first seen, it is usually a thin straw-coloured fluid. Later, it becomes thicker, more opaque and more distinctly yellow in colour. The nipple and its surrounding area (areola) become more deeply pigmented. This varies much in intensity in women of different complexions being more marked in darker than in fair-complexioned women. Small non-pigmented nodules appear on the areola, consisting of enlarged sebaceous glands. The areola becomes more prominent, and around it

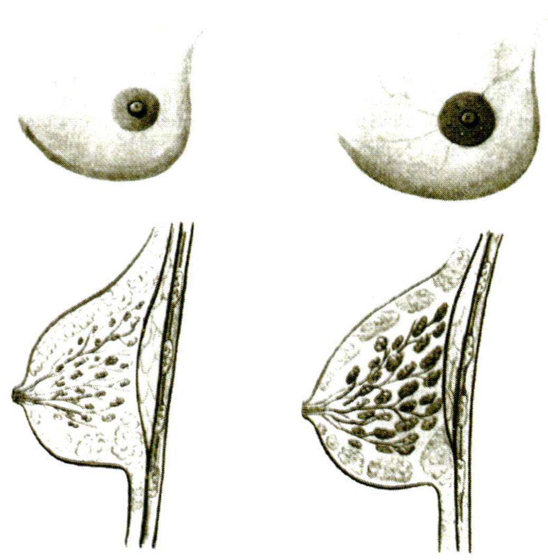

is formed an outer zone of irregular and less marked pigmentation known as the secondary areola. An increased blood flow, indicated by dilated veins under the skin accompanies the enlargement.

Enlargement of the belly

Enlargement of the belly usually takes long to show up. It becomes visible only when the uterus rises well above the pubes, and therefore seldom attracts attention until the close of the first half of pregnancy. A woman who has been pregnant earlier notices abdominal enlargement earlier than a first-time pregnant mother owing to her relatively lax abdominal wall.

Quickening

This term means 'coming to life' and indicates that the mother has become aware of the existence of something which is alive and moving within her. These initial movements of the baby felt by the mother sometimes produce a sensation of faintness. This is termed as 'quickening'. Many women do not experience it and find it impossible to tell when they first experienced the movements of the foetus. Mostly, they are first noticed between the 18th and the 20th week. The foetal movements continue until the end of pregnancy and are chiefly important in the later months as an indication that the baby is alive. The mother continues to be conscious of these movements and if she feels that they have stopped, she must immediately see her doctor.

It is usually with these symptoms that a woman decides to go to a doctor, to check whether she is pregnant. The doctor can sometimes confirm the pregnancy by an internal examination, but whenever there is a doubt the best and easiest way to confirm is by undertaking a pregnancy test.

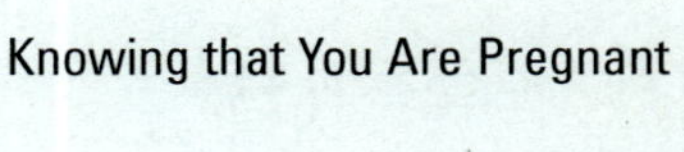

Tests to Confirm Pregnancy

Hormonal Tests

For a reliable pregnancy test, you have to wait until two weeks after the first day of a missed period. If you are pregnant, you would pass a sufficient amount of a particular pregnancy hormone (human chorionic gonadotrophin, or HCG for short) in the urine, which is readily detectable with the aid of a number of different tests. The easiest way is to collect the first urine passed in the morning and send it for testing to a close-by laboratory. Make sure that you collect the urine specimen in a clean, soap-free container, preferably one that has been provided by the lab.

You can also do the test at home. Just buy a do-it-yourself pregnancy testing kit, available with the chemist, follow the instructions given on the test kit and you have the result in no time. Make sure that you do the test carefully to fetch a reliable result.

The results of the test

You may ask, "how far can I rely on the results of this test?" If the test is done more than two weeks after your first missed period and if the result is positive, it is almost certainly right. Positive results are correct 99 times out of 100. On the other hand, if the result is negative, you cannot still be absolutely sure that you are not pregnant. It may be that there is not enough pregnancy hormone in the urine to show up in a test. If you still do not start a period have another test done in a week's time when it will be more reliable.

Ultrasound

In case the issue is still not resolved, a pelvic ultrasound done on full bladder can easily confirm or exclude the pregnancy. A normal ultrasound can pick a pregnancy as early as the fifth week (only a week after your period was due) and is almost cetain to do so at six

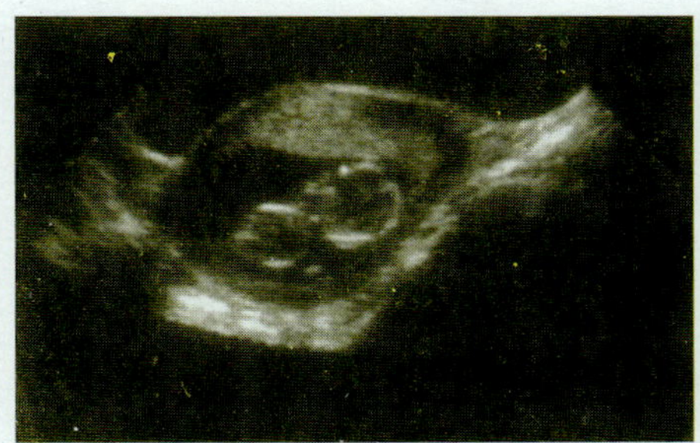

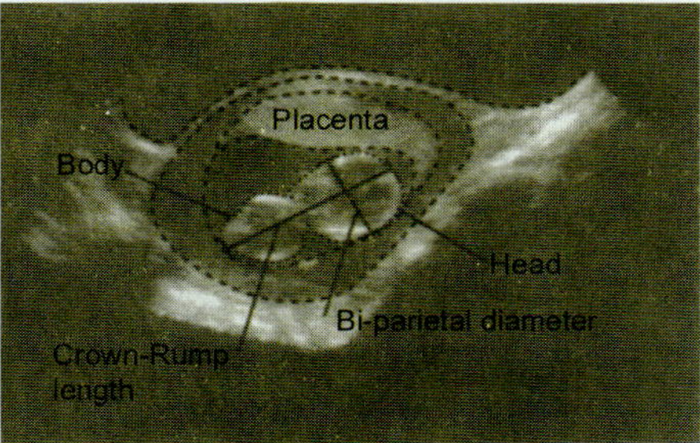

A 12-week pregnancy : That's how it looks on ultrasound

weeks. By the eighth gestational week, the embryo also becomes visible and its heart can be seen. The heart is in the middle of the growing embryo and is already beating to the life's rhythm.

The transvaginal ultrasound, which uses a special probe that is passed into the vagina, is quickest to detect the pregnancy.

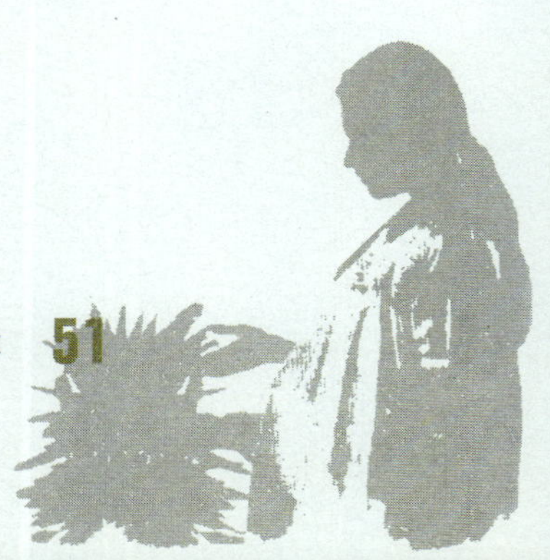

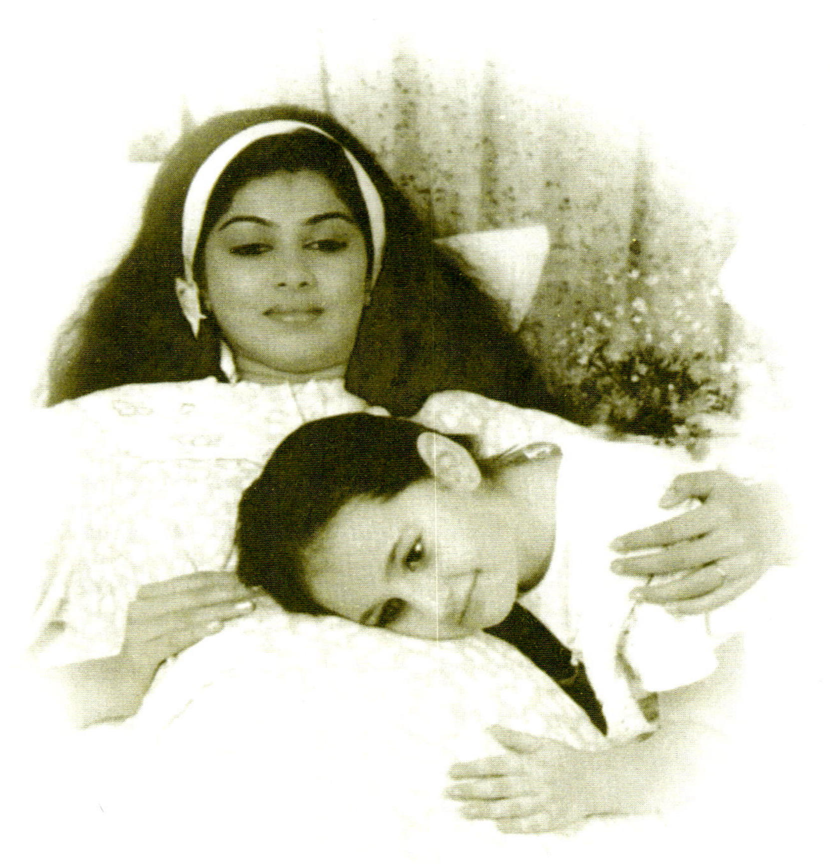

"A baby is God's opinion that life should go on."

-Carl Sandburg (1878-1967), U.S. poet.
Remembrance Rock.

The Exciting Happenings of Pregnancy

The birth of a playful independent-minded baby from a barely visible dot (the fertilised egg) 40-weeks ago is nothing short of a miracle. But that is exactly what makes a mother, a mother! Capable of nourishing the baby's development and growth with her own food and oxygen, she gives the fertilised egg her best from the very moment it develops its roots and links up with her.

A pregnancy begins with the fertilisation of the ovum. But doctors, for want of a better method, always time pregnancy from the first day of a woman's last monthly period. So what is considered 'four weeks pregnant', is actually about two weeks after conception. It is on this basis that a pregnancy lasts for 280 days. During this period a host of exciting changes take place. The baby develops and grows at a rapid pace and the mother goes through several remarkable changes.

How your baby develops

Here is a week-by-week summary of how your baby grows within you. Read on. It is truly exciting how 'your millimetres' shape into that bundle of joy!

Weeks 4-5

The developing fertilised egg now settles into the womb lining. Its outer cells reach out like roots to link with the mother's blood supply. The inner cells split into three layers. Each of these layers will grow to be different parts of the baby's body. One layer becomes the brain and nervous system, the skin, eyes and ears. Another layer becomes the lungs, stomach and gut. The third layer becomes the heart, blood, muscles and bones.

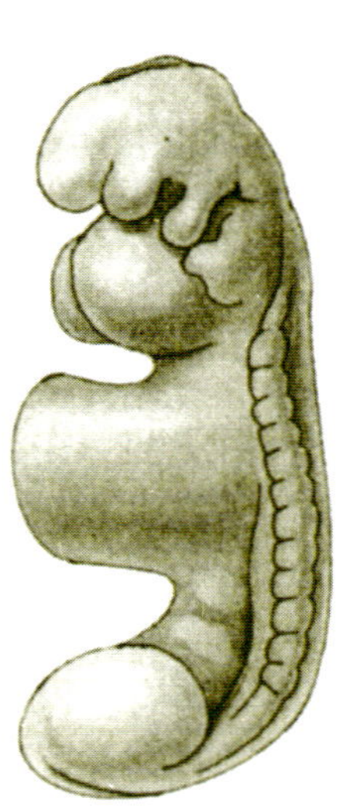

The fifth week is the time of the first missed period when most women are only just beginning to think they may be pregnant. Yet already the baby's nervous system is beginning to develop. A groove forms in the top layer of cells. The cells fold up and curl to make a hollow tube. This is called the neural tube. It will become the baby's brain and spinal cord, so the tube has a 'head end' and a 'tail end'. At the same time the heart is forming and the baby already has some of its own blood vessels. A string of these blood vessels connect baby and mother and will become the umbilical cord.

Weeks 6-7

There is now a large bulge where the heart is, and a bump for the head because the brain is developing. The heart begins to beat and can be seen beating in an ultrasound scan. Dimples on the side of the head will become the ears and there are thickenings where the eyes will be. On the body, bumps are forming which will become muscles and bones. Small swellings, called limb buds show where

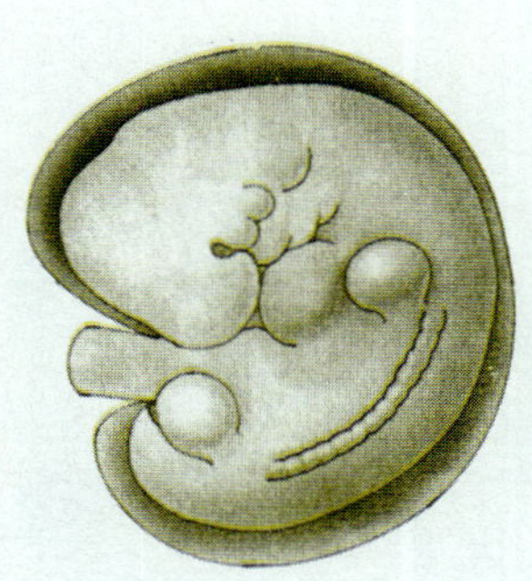

the arms and legs are growing. The lips and palate develop during the sixth to ninth weeks. Each forms from paired structures that gradually move from the sides toward the middle of the face and fuse. If anything interferes with normal development during this period, a split in the upper lip or palate may develop. Such a defect is called cleft lip or cleft palate.

At seven weeks the embryo is about 8 mm (1/3 inch) long from head to bottom or from crown to rump.

Weeks 8-9

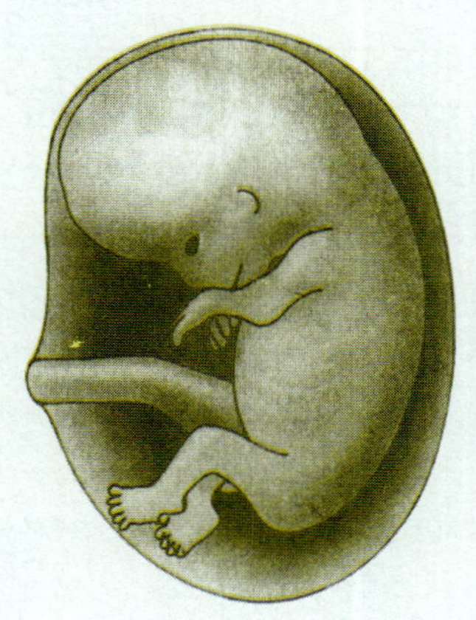

A face is slowly forming. The eyes are more obvious and have some colour in them. There is a mouth, with a tongue. There are now the beginnings of hands and feet with ridges where the fingers and toes will be. The major internal organs are all developing–the heart, brain, lungs, kidneys, liver and gut.

At nine weeks, the baby is about 17 mm (¾ inch) long from head to bottom.

Weeks 10-14

Just 12 weeks after conception, the foetus is fully formed. It has all its organs, muscles, limbs and bones. From now on it has to grow and mature.

The sex organs are now well developed. A highly trained sonologist can pick them out with a fair amount of accuracy. The

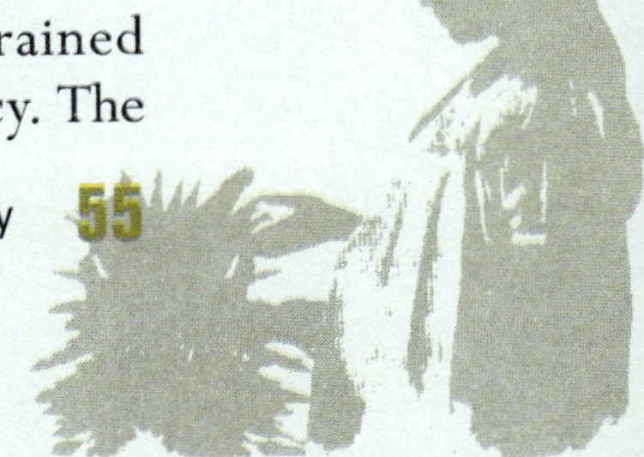

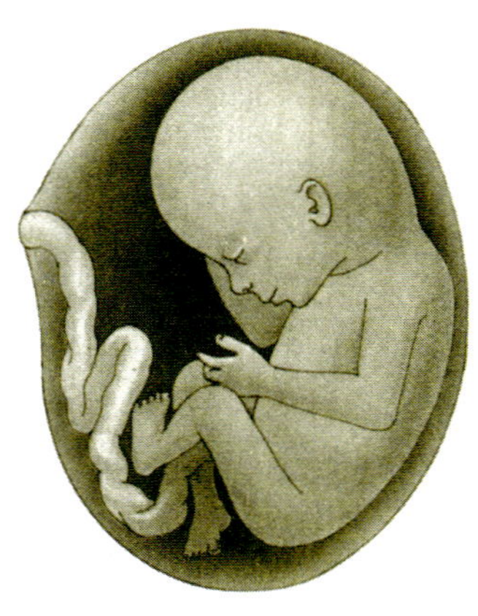

baby is already moving about but the movements cannot yet be felt.

By about 14 weeks the heartbeat is strong and can be heard using an ultrasound detector. The heartbeat is very fast, about twice as fast as a normal adult's heartbeat.

At 14 weeks the baby is about 56 mm (2¼ inches) long from head to bottom. The pregnancy may be just beginning to show, although this varies a lot from woman to woman.

Weeks 15-22

The baby is now growing quickly. The body grows bigger so that the head and body are more in proportion and the baby's head does not appear large. The face begins to look much more human and the hair begin to grow, as well as eyebrows and eyelashes. The eyelids stay closed over the eyes.

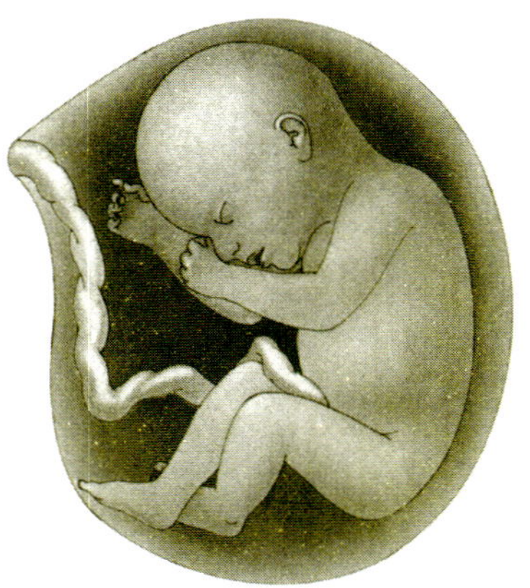

The lines on the skin of the fingers are now formed, so the baby already has its own individual fingerprint. Finger and toenails are growing, and the baby has a firm handgrip.

At about 22 weeks, the baby becomes covered in a very fine, soft hair called lanugo. The purpose of this is not known, but it is thought that it may be to keep the baby at the right temperature. The lanugo disappears before birth though sometimes just a little is left and disappears later.

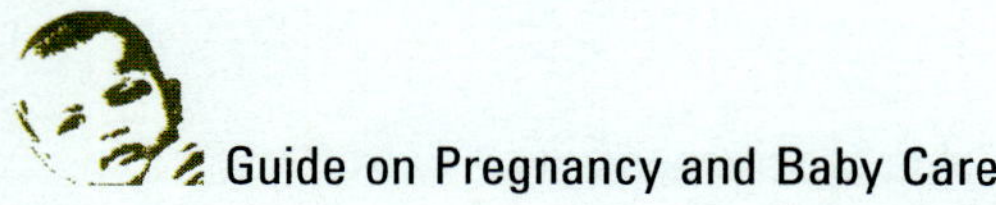

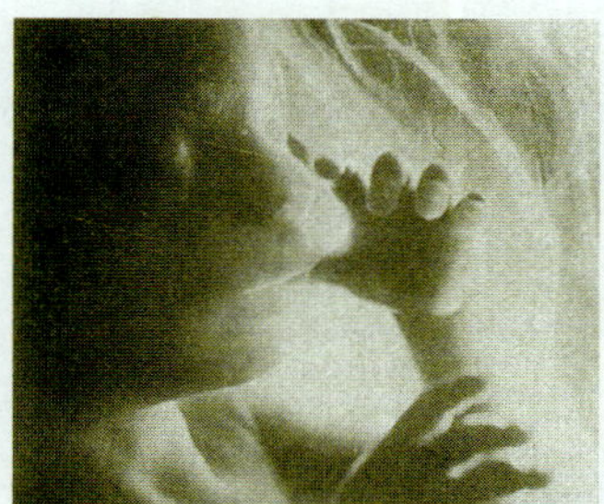

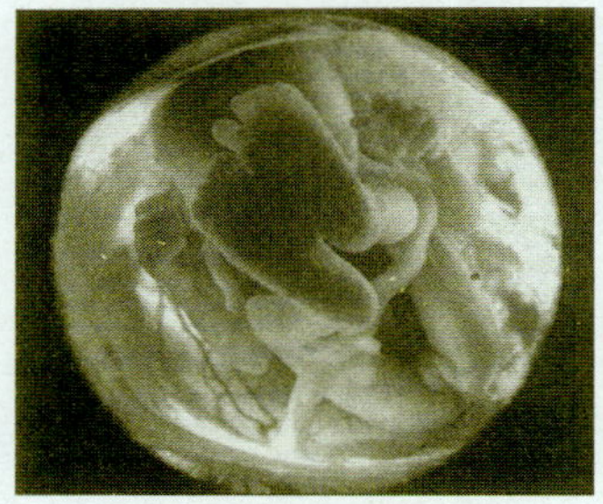

At about 18-20 weeks you will feel your baby move for the first time. If this is your second baby, you may feel it earlier at about 14 or 16 weeks after conception. At first you feel a fluttering or bubbling or a very slight shifting movement, maybe a bit like indigestion. Later you can't mistake the movements and you can even see the baby kicking about. Often you can guess which bump is a hand or a foot, and so on. Make a note of the date when you first feel your baby movement and tell the doctor. The date can be used to check your expected date of delivery.

At 22 weeks, the head to bottom length is about 160mm (6½ in).

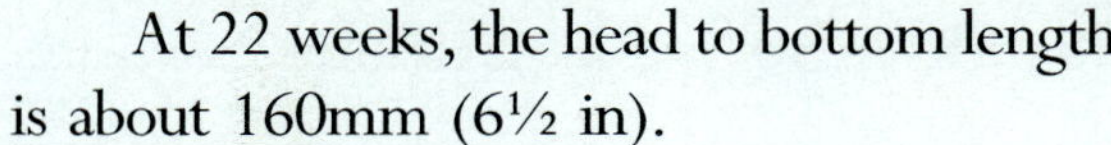

Weeks 23-30

The baby is now moving about vigorously and responds to touch and sound. A very loud noise close by may make it jump and kick. It swallows small amounts of the amniotic fluid in which it is floating and passes tiny amounts of urine back into the fluid. Sometimes the baby may get hiccups and you can feel the jerk of each hiccup. The baby may also begin to follow a pattern for waking and sleeping. Very often this is a different pattern from yours so when you go to bed at night, the baby wakes up and starts kicking.

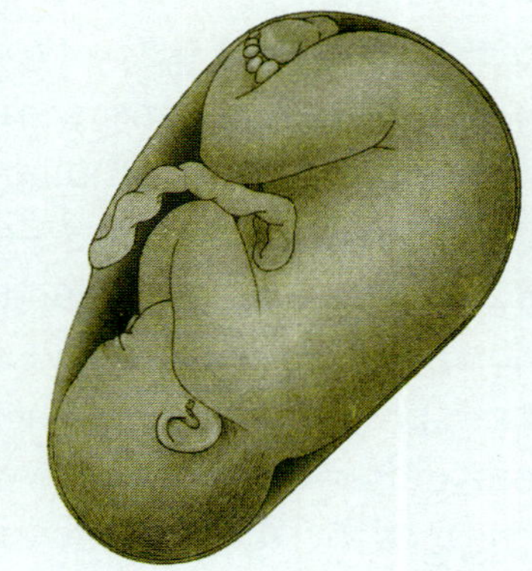

The baby's heartbeat can now be heard through a stethoscope. Your spouse may even be able to hear it by putting an ear to your belly, but he has to choose the right place!

The baby is now covered in a white, greasy substance called vernix. This protects the baby's skin as it floats in the amniotic fluid. The vernix mostly disappears before birth.

At around 26 weeks the baby's eyelids open for the first time. By the 28th week, the fingernails and toenails are well developed.

At 28 weeks, the baby is called 'viable'. This means that the baby is now thought to have a good chance of survival if born. Most babies born before this time cannot live because their lungs and other vital organs are not well developed. But if the baby can be placed in an incubator in a nursery with round-the-clock care in an intensive care neonatology unit, it may stand a chance.

The head to bottom length at 30 weeks is about 240 mm (9½ inches).

Weeks 31-40

Until the 30th week of pregnancy, the baby appears reddish and transparent because of the thinness of its skin and lack of fat beneath the skin. In the last six to eight weeks before birth, fat develops rapidly and the baby becomes smooth and plump. Both the vernix and the lanugo begin to disappear. By about 32 weeks the baby usually takes a head downwards position ready for birth. In a first time pregnant mother, the baby's head usually move down into the pelvis and becomes well engaged by the 36th week and remains well

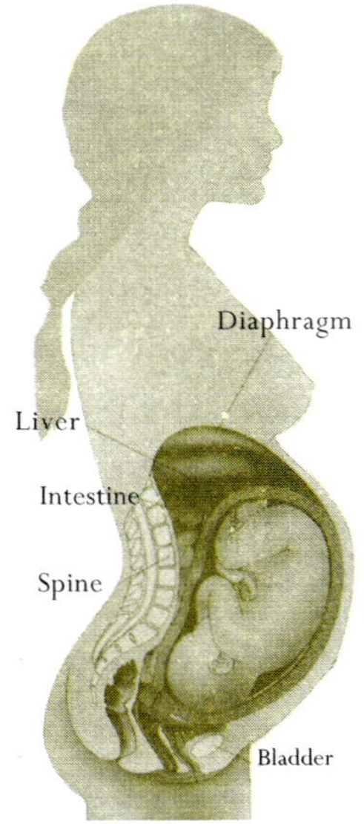

engaged from that date onwards. If it is still above the pelvic brim, the obstetrician likes to check out if the head can be pushed into the pelvic cavity. Otherwise, an elective Caesarean section may be necessary.

Nourishment for your baby

Various structures develop in the uterus to help the baby grow. These structures include the placenta and certain membranes. By the 13th day of pregnancy, a cavity-like space forms around the embryo. Two membranes surround this cavity. The outer membrane is called the chorion and the inner membrane is called the amnion.

The chorion interacts with tissues of the uterus to form the placenta. It pushes into the wall of the uterus with finger-like projections (chorionic villi), which contain the baby's first blood vessels. The chorion is attached to the baby by a structure called the body stalk. The body stalk develops into the umbilical cord which joins the baby to the placenta.

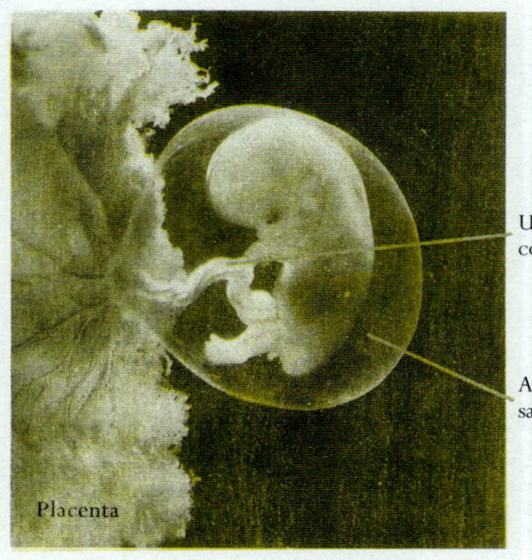

The amnion forms a sac around the baby and is filled with fluid. The baby floats in this fluid called amniotic fluid. The amniotic fluid protects the baby by absorbing jolts to the uterus. It also allows the baby to move without damaging the amnion and other tissues.

About the 21st day of pregnancy, blood begins to circulate between the placenta and the baby. The blood vessels of the mother

and those of the baby exchange substances through a thin layer of cells called the placental barrier. Waste products from the baby are carried away through the barrier. Likewise, nutrients and oxygen from the mother's blood pass through the thin walls of the barrier and enter the baby's blood. But, harmful organisms such as viruses and bacteria, chemical substances, and drugs which can harm the baby also sometimes breach the placental barrier.

Chromosomes and genes

Both the mother's egg and the father's sperm contain tiny, thread-like structures called chromosomes. It is through the chromosomes that characteristics like hair and eye colour, looks and build are passed from parents to child and it is the chromosomes that determine the baby's sex.

The fertilised egg contains 46 chromosomes, 23 from the mother and 23 from the father. Two of these chromosomes, one from the mother and one from the father are the sex chromosomes. The sex chromosome from the mother's egg is always the same and is called the X chromosome. But the sex chromosome from the father's sperm may be an X or a Y chromosome. If the egg is fertilised by a sperm containing an X chromosome then the baby will be a girl (XX). If the egg is fertilised by a sperm containing a Y chromosome then the baby will be a boy (XY).

There are only two ways of knowing your baby's sex before birth. Amniocentesis is a special test offered to only some women. It is used to detect certain abnormalities, but it also reveals the baby's sex. An ultrasound scan, if done at around 14th week of pregnancy or later may also show the baby's sex. But neither of these tests is legal unless there are definite medical reasons to check out the baby's sex for ruling out a serious sex-linked genetic defect.

The X and Y chromosomes and the other 44 chromosomes in the fertilised egg determine all the baby's inherited characteristics. Each chromosome carries about 2,000 genes and it is the genes which determine such things as the baby's blood group, height and build and hair and eye colour. The genes also influence characteristics like personality and intelligence, although these are affected by other things too, such as the environment a child gets.

Twins and Triplets

Identical twins are the result of one fertilised egg splitting into two separate cells. Each cell grows into a baby. Because they originally came from the same cell, the babies have the same genes. They are the same sex and look like each other. Non-identical twins are more common. They are the result of two eggs being fertilised by two sperm at the same time. The babies may not be of the same sex and will probably look no more alike than a brother and sister.

Twins are quite common. One in every 100 pregnancies results in twins. A couple is more likely to have twins if there is a history of twins from the mother's side. It is usually possible to find out if you are expecting twins by about the end of the second month of your pregnancy. An ultrasound scan can indicate that rather easily.

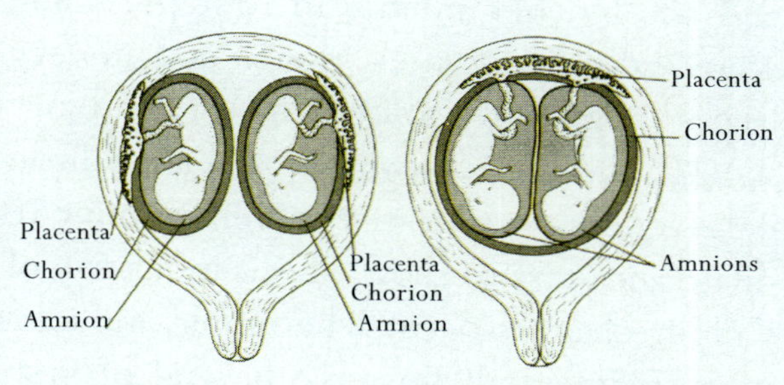

Non-identical Twins   Identical twins

Triplets are much more rare and quadruplets rarer still. Although nowadays the use of drugs in the treatment of infertility has made multiple births a bit more common, generally triplets are born once in every 8,100 pregnancies and quadruplets once in 7,29,000 pregnancies.

Changes A Mother Goes Through

A woman must go through a number of changes in her body during pregnancy. You would gain weight, the breasts would increase in size, the uterus would enlarge to accommodate the baby, the blood composition and volume would change, the endocrine organs would work overtime and the body would experience many changes in its functions.

Breasts

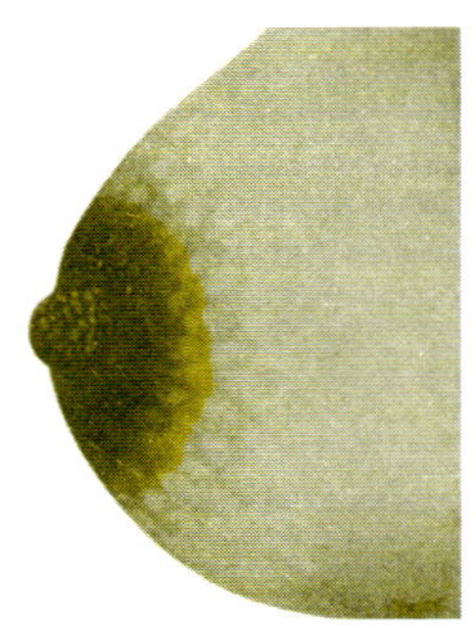

During the first pregnancy a woman's breasts undergo a series of changes. Many of these changes persist for life. The breasts are never fully developed until a woman has been pregnant and has fed her infant. In first pregnancy the whole gland increases in size and undergoes a hypertrophy. By about the second or third month, the breast begins to release a little clear pale-yellow secretion. The veins under its skin dilate and start to show. This is indicative of an increased blood flow. Colour changes occur. The nipple and its surrounding area become more pigmented. Towards the end of first pregnancy the skin over the breasts becomes stretched and develops linear streaks.

The breasts distend with milk three or four days following childbirth. Unless the baby is put to breast and the breasts are emptied, they become swollen and painful. A mother who is unable to feed her baby must empty the breasts mechanically to escape complications.

Milk is formed in the breasts due to hormonal stimulation. This hormone, prolactin, is released by the anterior lobe of the pituitary. The draught reflex set up during suckling enhances the flow of milk in the breast.

Skin

A woman undergoes several skin changes during pregnancy. While some are mechanical due to stretching of the skin, others are biological, like increase in pigmentation. Due to the increase in size, the belly develops linear stretch marks. In the beginning, they are pearly or pinkish in colour. Their size is variable and they are most marked below the navel. But sometimes they also appear on the adjacent parts of the buttocks and thighs. After the baby's birth their colour changes and they become pale and silvery. Not all pregnant women develop these marks. If the skin is very elastic, they may not appear at all.

As the pregnancy advances, several changes in pigmentation also occur. The face can develop irregular dark brown patches. These are most marked on the mother's forehead, the sides of the nose and the upper lip, but her whole face may be affected. It is called the pregnancy mask. The nipple and the surrounding areolae in the breasts also take a darker colour. During the second half of pregnancy, a thick dark line appears on the belly. It runs from above the navel to the pubes in the midline. Its colour varies with the complexion of the woman. It is usually broad and dark in a dark complexioned woman, but in fair women it may barely be visible. A similar line can also sometimes be seen in dark-complexioned women who have never been pregnant. Extensive pigmentation sometimes also occurs on the trunk in irregular patches, alternating with patches from which the natural pigment has largely disappeared.

These pigmentation changes disappear after childbirth, but sometimes, on the trunk, they become permanent.

Circulation

During pregnancy two major changes occur. One, the heart increases its output. Two, there is an increase in the blood volume. The resting output of the heart increases by about 40 per cent by the end of the first trimester. Subsequently, a further small increase may occur in the second trimester. After the 30th or 32nd week the heart's output is dependent on the mother's posture. If she reclines on one side the increased output is maintained till the baby is born but if she lies straight, the return of blood to the heart gets restricted due to obstruction of the big vein (inferior vena cava) by the pregnant uterus. This causes the supine output to fall in the last eight to 10 weeks. It is this sluggishness in flow which shows up in the form of piles, varicose veins of the legs and vulva and slight swelling of the feet. The normal heart meets the increased load of pregnancy without difficulty by encroaching slightly on its reserve power but this does not restrict the activity of the pregnant woman.

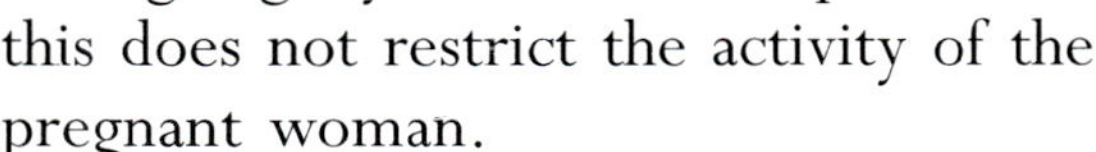

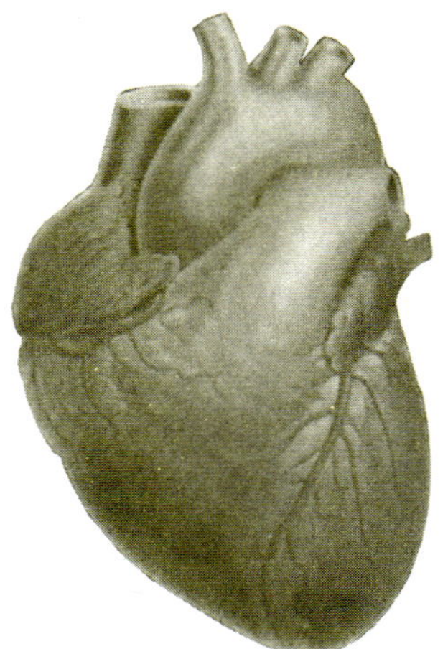

The blood volume increases from the 10th week and reaches a maximum at the 32nd week. The overall increase is about 30 per cent but the fluid element (plasma volume) increase is relatively greater than the increase in the red cell volume. This results in dilution of the red cells and a reduction in haemoglobin concentration. This dilutional anaemia is natural to pregnancy and should not raise any alarm. Often though, the situation gets complicated if the increased demands for iron and folic acid during pregnancy are not met. This worsens the anaemia.

The blood pressure in women of childbearing age normally ranges (in mm Hg) between 110 and 120 systolic and 65 and 80 diastolic. During pregnancy there is frequently a fall below these levels. Any pressure above 140 systolic and 90 diastolic should be regarded as abnormally high.

Endocrine glands

The thyroid enlarges during pregnancy and may become so large that it can be felt and seen as a swelling. The blood concentration of its hormone, thyroxine, rises. If the mother is iodine deficient, the burden of pregnancy may lead to obvious goitre formation.

The anterior pituitary also enlarges and becomes very vascular during pregnancy. So do the adrenals. The secretion of the adrenal hormone, cortisol, also therefore increases.

Urinary tract

The collecting system of the kidneys and the ureter, tubes that drain the kidneys, get dilated. This happens due to two factors: obstruction to the outflow of urine due to pressure of the pregnant uterus and lowering in muscular tone of the ureteral wall. This change is observed since the early weeks of pregnancy; it usually reaches its maximum about the middle of pregnancy, persists and may not subside completely until about 12 weeks after childbirth. The thing to remember is, if your ultrasound report mentions it, do not worry.

The bladder also usually shows some irritability about the second month, but this passes off and does not recur until the close of pregnancy, when micturition may again become frequent and uncomfortable.

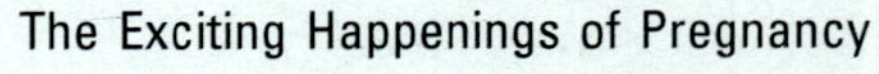

Changes in respiration

In the later half of pregnancy the enlarged uterus causes difficulty in the movement of the diaphragm. This causes some discomfort in respiration. The breathing movement becomes almost entirely dependant on the movement of the ribs. Due to increased needs and shallowness of effort, the rate of respiration becomes high.

Musculo-skeletal system

During the second month of pregnancy, the mother may frequently complain of cramps in the legs. These occur because of pressure upon the lumbar and sacral plexuses. In addition, the pelvic joints undergo slight softening of ligaments and general loss of firmness and strength. This may lead to backache. But if you are careful about your posture and body mechanics, you can find quick relief.

Changes in the general metabolism

Pregnancy is a state of harmonious symbiosis between the mother and the baby. The demands of the baby on mother's nutrition are certainly not overtaxing and have been described elsewhere in this book (see chapter five).

Changes in the level of the uterine height

The uterus rises as it grows in the mother's belly with each passing week. At 12 weeks it starts to edge above the symphysis, the front part of the bony pelvis. By 16 weeks, it rises to midway between the symphysis and the navel. It further rises to the level of the navel by about 22-24 weeks. About the 36th week the uterus attains its greatest height in the abdomen, extending nearly to the lower tip of the breastbone and the abdominal girth may reach 36 inches. During the last fortnight of pregnancy, it usually sinks by about an inch.

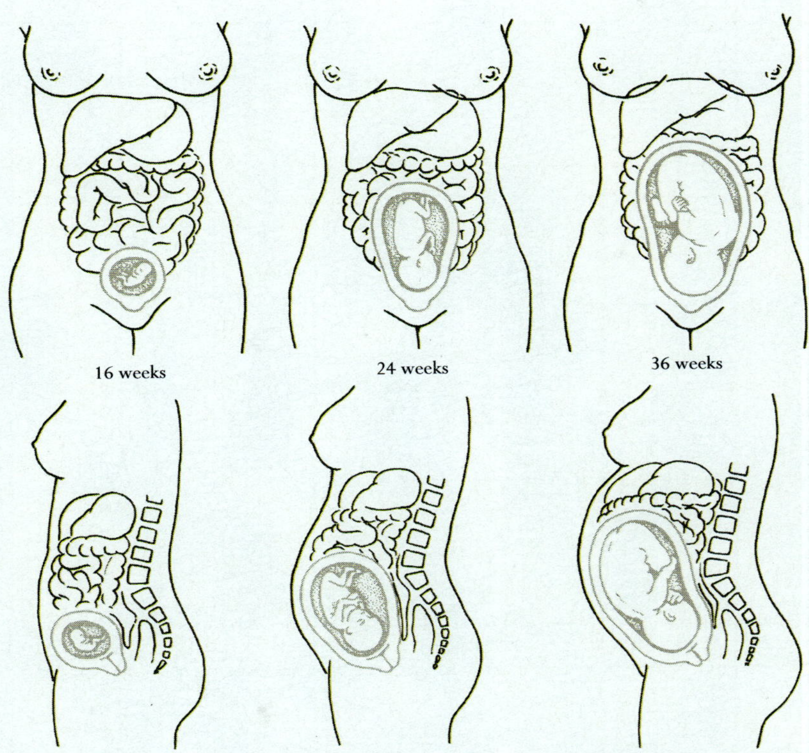

The height of the uterus is a good guide for the doctor. If the fundus is rising too rapidly or if it is not rising at the normally anticipated rate, it means that all is not well and an investigation may be required.

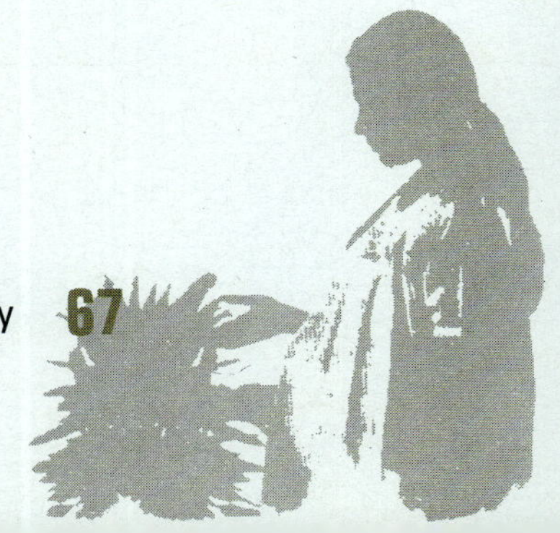

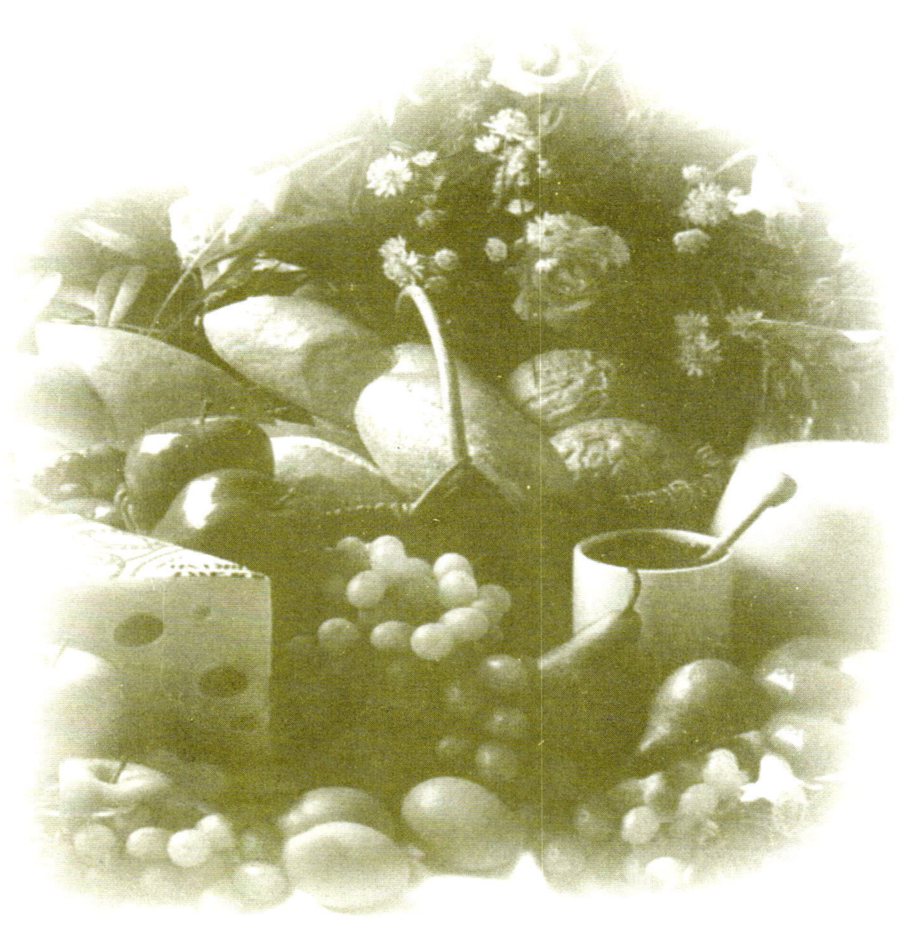

"A healthy diet is a fitting recipe for good health and your body, mind and brain to function well."

-Chandogya Upanishad

What to Eat and Why

Just as at all times the key to healthier pregnancy is to eat a well-balanced nutritious diet. You simply have to stick to the basic principles and guard against overdoing it. The notion that a pregnant woman must eat for two is all wrong and an idea of a bygone era. A balance of proteins, carbohydrates, fats and sufficient amounts of essential vitamins and minerals are ample for the mother-to-be and her baby. Health foods and the fat-rich dry fruit studded Indian flour recipe of "panjeeri" are certainly passé.

What should a pregnant mother eat? Much has been written and spoken about this. All kinds of well-meant advices offered but all that is needed is, to follow the basic rules of healthy eating. That alone would ensure your good health and that of the baby.

By making a healthy diet a habit even before you conceive, you increase your baby's chances of developing healthily and well. That is because the baby depends on you for food from the moment of conception.

Food is primarily made of carbohydrate, fat, proteins, vitamins, mineral and water. An expectant mother must eat a balanced diet to ensure good health.

Carbohydrates

Carbohydrates give us energy. They are necessary in adequate amounts to spare protein for growth. The main sources of carbohydrates are fruits, vegetables, confections and grain products. The unrefined sources have valuable fibre. Sweet confections also provide carbohydrates, but are often called "empty calories", because they do not have much nutritious value.

Fats

Fats are a concentrated source of energy, yielding over twice as many calories as carbohydrates. Besides supplying energy, fat in the diet provides essential fatty acids and supplies and carries the fat soluble vitamins, A, D, E, and K. Also, fats such as butter and vegetable oil add to the palatability of food.

Proteins

The main function of proteins is to build and repair all body cells. An increased amount is needed during pregnancy for growth and maintenance of maternal and baby's tissues. Proteins are made up of different combinations of the more than 20 amino acids. Eight of these cannot be synthesized by the body and are referred to as essential amino acids, which must be supplied by the diet. Proteins that contain adequate amounts of all the eight essential amino acids are called complete proteins. Most vegetable protein sources are deficient in one or more of the essential amino acids. The amino acids that are in short supply in any given protein are called limiting amino acids. The body can use the protein to the level of the limiting amino acid and what is left over is used for energy. Two or more "incomplete" protein sources with different limiting amino acids can be combined in the same meal and are then used as a complete protein. For instance, the amino acids in pulses easily supplement those in cereals. No wonder, the native dal-roti holds us in good stead!

Vitamins

Vitamins are vital to good health. They are organic substances that are essential and must be supplied by the diet in minute amounts daily. They are directly involved in regulating the metabolism of carbohydrate, protein, and fat and they assist in regulating reactions by which body tissues are maintained. Many reactions in the body require more than one vitamin and the lack of any one can interfere with the function of another. Most vitamins cannot be synthesised by the body. The human body can store fat-soluble vitamins and therefore large doses, especially of vitamins A and D can be toxic. Excesses usually come from excessive supplementation, not from food sources.

Vitamin A assists in maintaining the integrity of the mucous membrane, which increases the body's resistance to infection. It is also essential for normal bone growth and tooth development and plays a role in night vision. Carotene, which is synthesized by plants and is the usual form of the vitamin in foods, is the precursor of vitamin A. Dark green and deep yellow vegetables and fruits are the

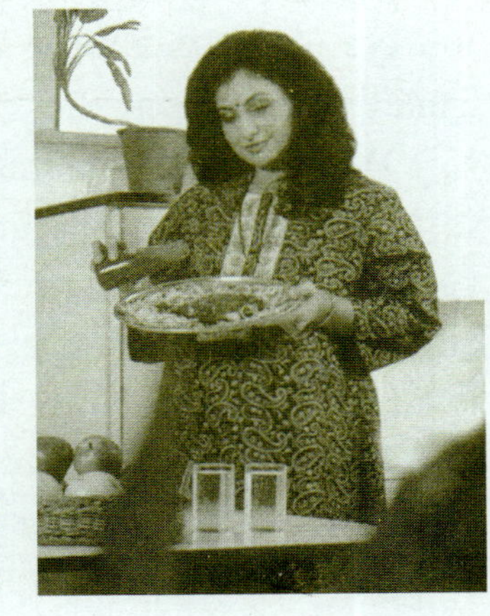

best sources of vitamin A. Milk and vanaspati oil also are good sources of vitamin A.

Vitamin D plays a role in the absorption and utilisation of calcium and phosphorus in bone and tooth bud formation. Egg yolk, liver, and certain fish contain fair amounts of vitamin D. Cod liver oil was used as a supplement for years to prevent rickets in children. To make vitamin D readily available, it is also added in vanaspati oil, butter and milk. The human body also produces some amounts due to the action of sunlight on the skin.

Vitamin E is primarily an antioxidant. It reduces oxidation of the polyunsaturated fatty acids, helping to maintain the integrity of the cell membranes. It is also involved in certain enzymatic and metabolic reactions. The main sources of vitamin E in the diet are vegetable fats and oils, leafy green vegetables, grains, nuts and egg yolks.

Vitamin K is an essential factor in the formation of prothrombin, and is therefore necessary for normal blood clotting. Leafy green vegetables, potatoes and pork liver are excellent dietary sources of this vitamin. Vitamin K is also synthesized naturally. Some friendly bacteria in the lower intestinal tract do that for us.

Water-soluble vitamins are not stored in any significant amount, so it is easier for deficiencies to develop than with the fat-soluble vitamins. The B complex group actually consists of a number of different vitamins that are essential to good nutrition. These include thiamine (vitamin B_1), riboflavin (vitamin B_2), niacin (vitamin B_6), folacin (folic acid), and cyanocobalamin (vitamin B_{12}). They act as components of enzymes and coenzymes in many reactions in the body, such as cell respiration, glucose oxidation, and energy metabolism. Requirements are increased to meet the increased metabolic and growth needs of pregnancy. The B vitamins are not all found together in the same foods; however, if the diet includes milk, whole grain or enriched cereals and breads, legumes and dark green vegetables, eggs, organ and other meats, most of them will probably be present. Vitamin B_{12} is only found in foods of animal origin.

Folic acid is one of the B vitamins. It is involved in deoxyribonucleic acid (DNA) and ribonucleic acid (RNA) synthesis. If there is a lack of folic acid, cell division cannot proceed normally. There is an increased need during pregnancy for growth of the baby and in expansion of maternal blood volume. Recent research has found that if a mother takes sufficient amount of folic acid in early pregnancy the risk of nervous system defects in the baby decreases significantly. Leafy green vegetables, other green vegetables, liver, yeast, legumes, nuts, and whole grains are sources of folic acid, but as much as 80 per cent of the vitamin may be destroyed in cooking or storage, so supplementation is often advised.

Vitamin C is essential for the formation of collagen, which is sometimes called the cement that holds the body's cells and tissues together. This helps to explain the importance of vitamin C in building strong bones and teeth, healing wounds and aiding the ability of the body to withstand the stresses of injury and infection. Vitamin C is found in fresh vegetables and fruits, especially citrus fruits. Fresh strawberries, cantaloupe, pineapple, guavas, tomatoes, and the green vegetables also are good sources. Other fruits and vegetables can be important dietary sources if eaten in sufficient quantity. Vitamin C is easily destroyed by exposure to air, overcooking or cooking in too much water.

Minerals

Minerals are also an essential part of good nutrition. Some of these are found in fairly large amounts in the body and others called trace elements or micronutrients, are found in minute amounts. Minerals are constituents of vital body materials and some act as regulators and activators of body functions.

Calcium is an important constituent of bone and teeth. It is also used by the body for other functions, such as normal blood clotting, promoting muscle tone and regulating the heartbeat. Although two thirds of the calcium in a baby is deposited during the last month of pregnancy, the mother's daily requirement of calcium increases during the entire course of pregnancy to meet the later requirement. The principal foods from which calcium is obtained are cheese, eggs, oatmeal, vegetables and milk. Two large glasses of milk alone supplies about 1200 mg of calcium.

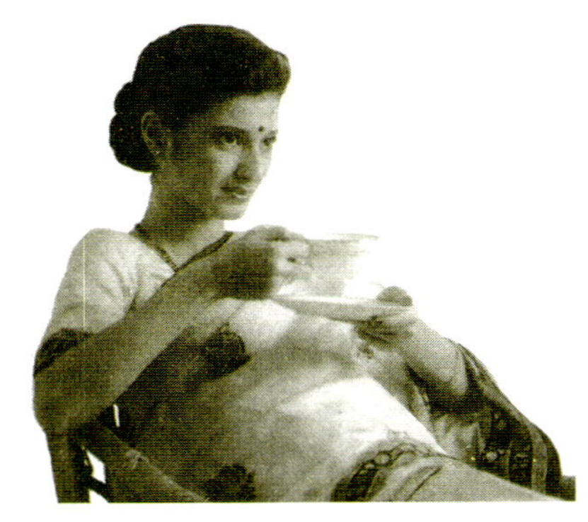

Phosphorus is an essential constituent of all the cells and the tissues of the body. Milk provides an abundant source of phosphorus. Phosphorus is an almost invariable constituent of protein, hence a diet which includes sufficient protein-rich foods such as, eggs, meat, cheese, oatmeal, and green vegetables, will provide an adequate amount of phosphorus.

Iron is one of the chief components of haemoglobin, the substance in the blood responsible for carrying oxygen to the cells. During pregnancy iron is needed to manufacture haemoglobin for baby's red blood cells as well as maternal red blood cells. During the first two trimesters of pregnancy, iron is transferred to the baby in moderate amounts, but during the last trimester, when the baby builds up its reserve, the amount transferred is accelerated about 10 times. The diet should therefore be rich in iron. The best way is to eat dark green leafy vegetables, jaggery (gur), peas, beans, nuts and dried apricots if you are a vegetarian or red meat, eggs and oysters if you are not such a stickler for grass. However, dietary sources of iron and limited maternal stores cannot supply the amounts needed for pregnancy. Therefore, supplementation of 30 mg to 60 mg of elemental iron, daily, is recommended. A glass of orange juice taken with iron can enhance absorption.

Iodine is needed in very small amounts by the pregnant mother and the baby. This mineral is obtained very readily from soil. In India, the soil is deficient in iodine and hence the water supply and the vegetables grown on the soil, do not fulfil the daily needs. Daily use of iodised salt ensures an adequate intake of iodine and prevents any deficiency.

Zinc also has an important role to play during pregnancy. If taken in sufficient amount, the risk of baby growing poorly during its intra uterine life is diminished. On the other hand, its deficiency has been linked to congenital malformations and delivery complications, including prolonged labour. Most protein foods—milk, fish and egg yolks have reasonable zinc content, so a diet meeting the daily requirement for protein should also furnish sufficient amounts of zinc.

Sodium is present in foods of animal origin, and in some vegetables, but the major dietary source is salt. There is an increasing emphasis on the importance of adequate sodium intake during pregnancy. In the past restriction on salt intake was thought to be an important factor in the prevention of toxaemia. Clinical and laboratory data now indicate that sodium requirement increases during pregnancy. Restriction, therefore, can be harmful when imposed indiscriminately. Many physicians now advise patients, early in the pregnancy to simply, "salt their food to taste." However, this does not mean that salt intake needs to be increased!

Water

Water is often omitted when nutrients are listed, but it is, a very essential nutrient. It constitutes two-thirds of the human body and is an important solvent necessary for digestion, nutrient transport to the cells and removal of body wastes. It is also a lubricant and helps regulate body temperature. Fluids should be taken freely, averaging six to eight glasses daily. Water and juices are good choices. Some other beverages contain ingredients that should be used sparingly in the prenatal diet. For example, regular soft drinks contain many empty calories, dietetic soft drinks contain artificial sweeteners, and cola, tea, and coffee contain caffeine. It makes sense to decrease their intake.

Supplements

Most obstetricians routinely prescribe vitamin and mineral supplements to all pregnant women. They feel it helps to be on the safe side. Others prescribe just iron and folacin, because these two nutrients are difficult to obtain adequately by diet alone. Other supplements may be needed in specific circumstances, such as calcium for the woman who drinks little or no milk and vitamin B_{12} for a vegetarian. If any vitamin or mineral supplements are used, it is important for the woman to understand that they are in addition to, not instead of her recommended dietary intake.

The popular notion that a pregnant woman should eat for two is a dangerous fallacy. You should eat moderately, for there is more harm in eating too much than too little. Overeating leads to obesity and digestive disturbances and there is evidence that it increases the liability to eclampsia and other toxaemias of pregnancy. Yet, most would-be-mothers in Indian homes are pampered and fed on high calorie foods. That is all wrong. What you need is simply an increase of 300 calories in the daily intake.

You could do so by simply increasing your milk intake to 600 ml day, eating a piece of cheese three or four times in a week, taking dal or meat, fish and eggs on a regular basis and enjoying sufficient amounts of fresh fruits and vegetables in your diet. This will ensure adequate supply of the nutrients you and your baby need the most.

Weight Watching

It is most important that you do not gain extra weight during pregnancy. The total gain for the entire length of pregnancy should

Additional Dietary Allowances During Pregnancy

Food items	How Much Extra You Need	Calories provided (kcal)
Cereals	35 gram	118
Pulses	15 gram	52
Milk	100 gram	83
Fat	—	—
Sugar	10 gram	40
Total		293

Source: Recommended dietary intakes for Indians: Indian Council of Medical Research

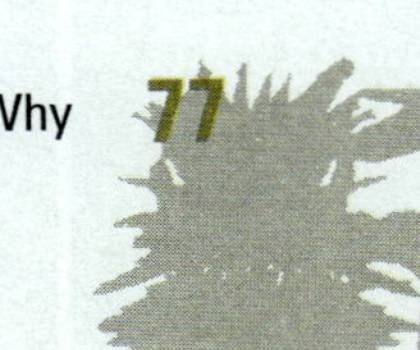

DIET PLAN FOR A PREGNANT MOTHER

[Approximate calories—2200]

Suitable for a mother who weighs 48kg

7 a.m.	Tea-1 cup; Dates- 5 or 6 pieces; and 2 or 3 Marie biscuits or Suji ka rusk
8.30 a.m.	Bread slices (2 pieces) or porridge (1 bowl) or idli (2 pieces) or chapatis – 2 with vegetable (1 katori); Cheese –1 piece or one egg; and Milk –1glass
11 a.m.	Seasonal fruit or roasted chana (1 bowl) or sprouts (1 bowl)
1p.m.	Chapatis 3 or 4 (medium sized) or Rice (3 scoops) Dal – 1 katori Green vegetable – 1 katori Curd – 1 bowl Salad – 1 plate
4 p.m.	Milk shake (1 glass) or cheese sandwich (1 small) or poha or upma (1 serving)
8.30 p.m.	Chapatis 3 or 4 (medium sized) or Rice (3 scoops) Dal –1 katori Green vegetable – 1 katori Curd – 1 bowl Paneer or meat or fish or chicken – 1 bowl Salad – 1 plate
9.30 p.m.	Milk (1 glass)

Calorie intake calculated as per the Indian Council of Medical Research guidelines
Calorie need=40 calories per kg body weight
Extra allowance for pregnancy=300 calories

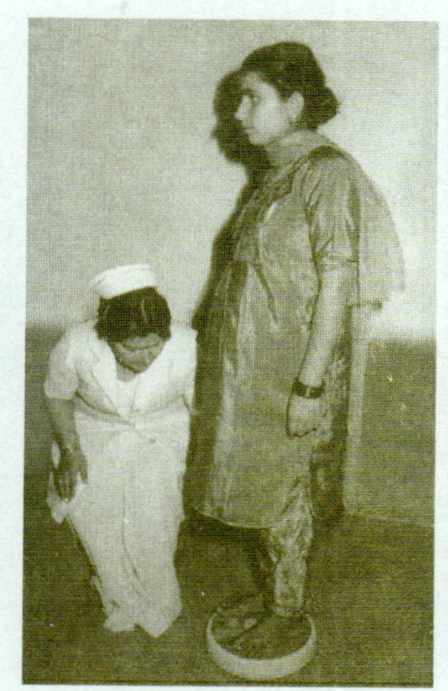

not be more than 10 or 12 kilos. Many studies have shown that both too much or too less gain in weight carries risks. If the mother's weight is static or falling, there is a real risk that the baby will be of low birth weight and have an increased risk of intrauterine death. In contrast, excessive increase in weight increases in the mother the risk of toxaemia in the present state and in later life lead to obesity with all its complications.

The fat deposits in pregnancy are mainly around the lower trunk and upper thighs. It gets laid down particularly in the middle trimester. The hormone, progesterone, encourages the accumulation. The reason for the storage is to provide a readily available energy bank should the mother not be able to take sufficient food.

You must however always avoid an unnecessary gain in weight. Limit high calorie foods which contain little or no protein, minerals and vitamins. Fried foods, cream, sweets, chocolates, sugar, glucose, cakes, pastries, puddings and biscuits, jam, marmalade, honey and most junk foods are simply avoidable. If despite these restrictions you experience excessive gain in weight, consult your doctor. A gain of over 0.5 kilos in a week should ring an alarm.

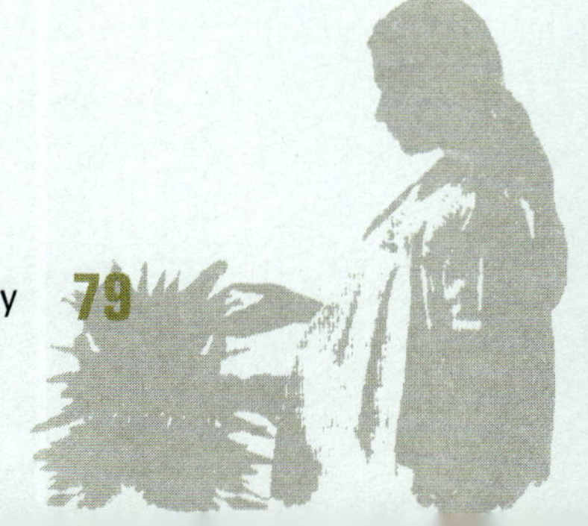

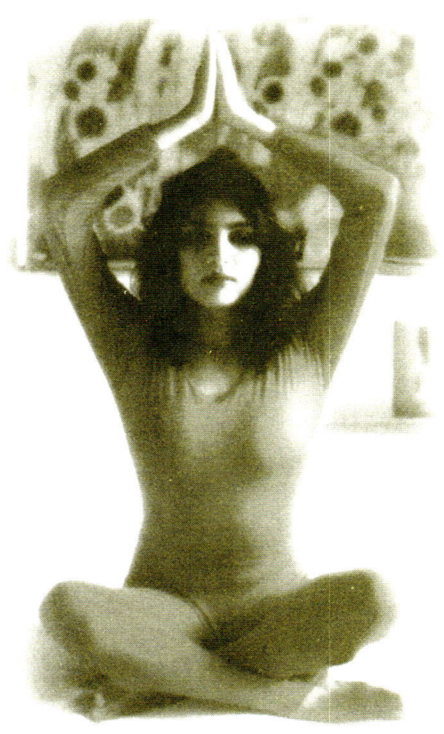

*"The preservation of health is a duty.
Few seem conscious that there is such a thing
as physical morality."*

-Herbert Spencer (1820-1903), English philosopher.
Education.

How Simple Asanas and Exercises Help

Maintaining correct posture and practicing good body mechanics are important in avoiding some of the more common discomforts of pregnancy. As the pregnant mother's centre of gravity is gradually shifted forward, the body frame is put to definite strain. But if she is mindful of her posture, maintains a correct body alignment and distributes the excess weight and stress efficiently and evenly she can avoid straining herself. Some easy exercises can also train her muscles and ligaments and she can breathe more easily and in rhythm during childbirth.

As you nurture your baby within you, your body goes through definite changes. By the fourth month, your body proportion and weight distribution have begun to change. The body's centre of gravity shifts forward, the abdominal muscles relax and the natural curvature of the spine becomes exaggerated, shortening the muscles of the lower back. You try to balance yourself by leaning backward slightly at the waist, but this shifts your weight to your heels when walking. You end up sporting an awkward, waddling gait and develop a backache. Yet if you are a little careful and mindful of your posture, take care as to how you stand, sit, climb stairs and carry packages or lift objects, you could easily escape these pains and aches. Good posture and body mechanics and exercises to reinforce muscles and joints can protect you from undue strain. This will enable you to carry on with your activities all during pregnancy.

Maintain good body alignment

To get the feel of good body alignment, stand with your feet about 10 inches away from the wall and press your hips, spine and the back of your head against the wall. Take a deep breath, exhale and relax and try to gain a sense of your body alignment as you stand in this position. You can also take a cue on the common mistakes we all make and how they can be corrected by looking at the checklist below.

Incorrect Posture

Head

Neck sags, chin pokes forward and whole body slumps

Shoulders and chest

Slouching cramps the rib cage and makes breathing difficult
Arms turn in

Abdomen and buttocks

Slack muscles cause a hollow back
Pelvis tilts forward

Knees

Pressed back knees strain joints and push pelvis forward

Correct Posture

Head

Straighten neck and tuck chin in so body lines up

Shoulders and chest

Lift up through rib cage and pull shoulder girdle back
Roll arms out

Abdomen and buttocks

Contract abdominal to flatten back
Tilt buttocks under and tilt pelvis back

Knees

Bend to ease body weight over feet

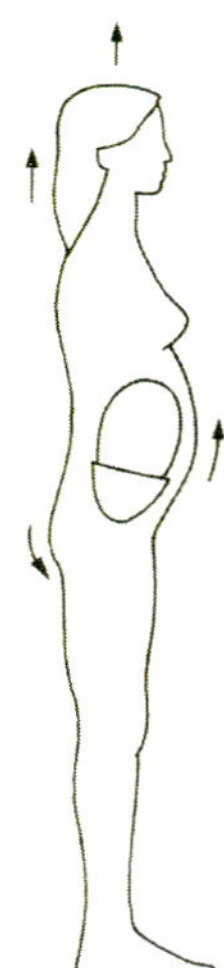

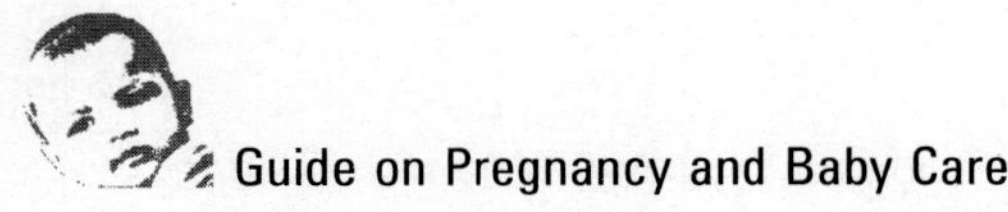

The healthy way of doing things

You must also learn the importance of practicing good body mechanics. This involves the efficient use of the body to evenly distribute weight and stress among several muscle groups rather than overtaxing a particular muscle group with undue strain. Here are a few simple do's and don'ts:

- You should shift position and do different activities at short intervals. For instance, walking back and forth is preferable to standing still. This way you use different group of muscles each time and the load is more evenly shared.
- Stand with one leg forward. This will allow you the opportunity of shifting your weight easily and efficiently from foot to foot and you can turn the body comfortably.
- Walk with head erect, back upright, chin up and pelvis tilted.
- Use a footstool while sitting.
- While climbing stairs, place the entire foot on the stair and use leg muscles to lift self up, each step, without leaning forward.
- Avoid stooping and lifting. Bending forward or stooping may put you off balance. It will strain the muscles of the back when you finally straighten yourself. If stooping is necessary, it is best to squat down and reach and lift, with feet wide apart and back straight. You should pull the object to be lifted close to the body and use the muscles of the thighs and legs to raise yourself up.
- When you need to carry bulky packages such as groceries, divide the load and carry it in two hands.

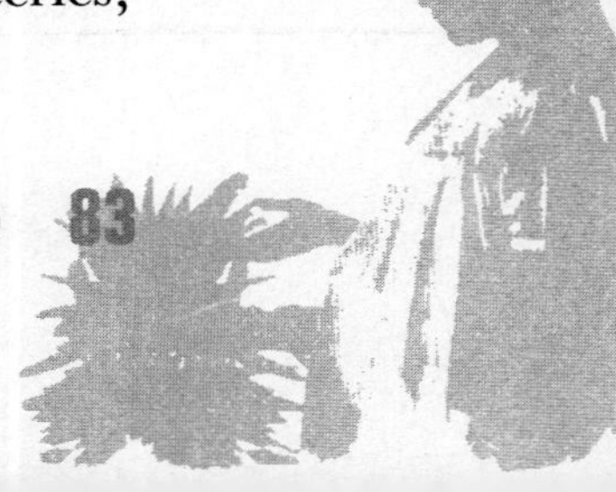

Relax with simple asanas

A variety of positions have been found effective in providing comfort and in relieving some of the discomforts of pregnancy. They could relieve you of backache, fatigue, swelling, cramps, and a number of other discomforts. Let us take a quick look at these positions and the benefits they offer.

Use this position to relax

Sit on the floor with your knees spread as far apart as comfortable, with one leg resting on the floor in front of the other and the back straight. Rest your back against a wall or take some other support. This will make it more comfortable. Begin by keeping this position for about five minutes at a time and gradually increase to intervals of 15 minutes to 30 minutes. This position significantly decreases circulation to the legs and feet; you should therefore shake out your legs every few minutes and then return to the position.

This is a good position to relax. It helps in stretching the muscles of the thighs, hips, and lower back and is therefore helpful in finding relief from lower backache.

Raise the legs against a wall

Lie straight on the bed. Now raise the legs taking the support of a wall by resting your heels against it. Hold for two to five minutes. Repeat several times each day making necessary adjustments suiting the stage of pregnancy. For instance, in early pregnancy, the body and legs can be nearly at a right angle with the buttocks against the wall or very close to it. However, as pregnancy advances, the right-

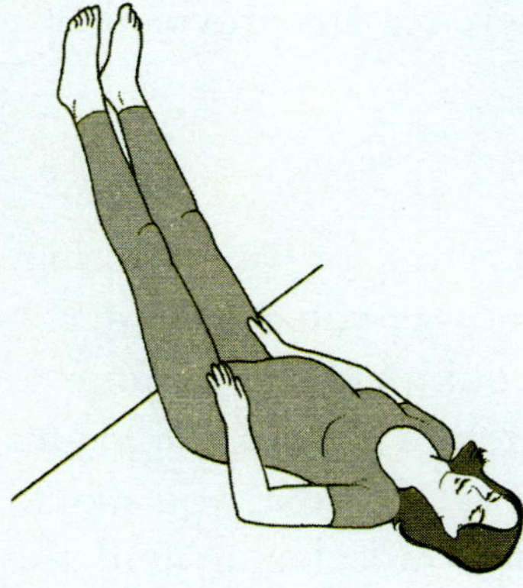

angle position becomes uncomfortable because of pressure on the diaphragm. You may therefore move your body slightly away from the wall to reduce the angle. Relax for a few moments after lowering your legs and rise slowly.

This is an easy method of improving circulation in the legs. It also gives relief from fatigue, swelling, cramps and varicose veins of the legs.

Try the knee-chest position

Turn on your stomach and raise your body so that your knees and chest are close together. The chest should be against the floor and the knees should be about a foot apart. Hold this position for about two minutes.

The knee-chest position is effective in relieving lower back pain. It is also helpful in relieving the discomforts of piles, swelling around the vagina, cramps in the thighs and buttocks and heaviness in the pelvis.

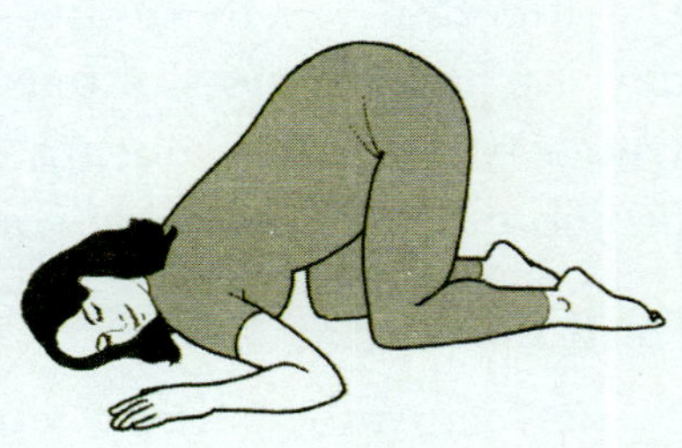

Some easy fitness exercises

You can improve circulation, enhance muscle tone, increase physical comfort and avoid fatigue by doing some simple exercises during pregnancy. Always do them smoothly avoiding jerky movements. Never do any exercise that causes pain or discomfort. Some obstetric care centres offer special exercise classes for pregnant and postpartum women. A group setting is often helpful because

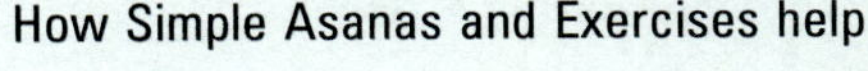

motivation is enhanced. The following exercises are provided as a general guide.

Pelvic floor exercises

You can do this simple exercise in a standing, sitting or lying position. Just draw up the muscles of the pelvic floor as you would if you were attempting to avoid urinating. You would feel the squeeze as the muscles surrounding the vagina and urethra tighten. Hold this tightness for two or three seconds and then relax. Next, you should perform the same exercise, tightening the muscles around the rectum and eventually tightening all of the muscles of the perineum at the same time. You should progress to doing 50 or more pelvic floor contractions each day, holding each contraction for five seconds.

These exercises help relieve the feeling of heaviness in the pelvis and give you better urinary control, preventing it from leaking during an activity or while coughing or laughing. They also strengthen and increase the flexibility of the pelvic floor muscles and help develop an awareness of tension and relaxation in the perineal area, which is important during childbirth. After childbirth, they help promote healing, provide comfort, and to help regain muscle tone.

Pelvic tilt exercise

To perform this exercise you should be on hands and knees, with hands directly under the shoulders and the knees under the hips. The back should be in a neutral position with the small of the back flattened, not hallowed. Your head and neck should be aligned with a straight back and your elbows and knees should remain stationary. Now pull in the abdominal muscles and

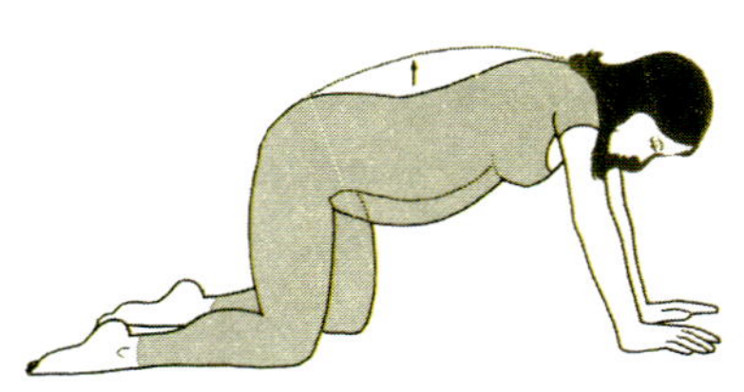

buttocks and press up with your lower back. Hold this position for a few seconds. Relax in the neutral position. Repeat five times, maintaining a slow rhythmic motion. Initially, you may need assistance in assuming the neutral position and avoiding a sagging or hollow back posture.

The pelvic tilt exercise is useful in strengthening the muscles of the abdomen and the lower back. It is thus helpful in relieving backache. It may also be used during a labour to relieve backache and to help in rotating the baby's head when the presentation is posterior.

Stretch the calf muscles

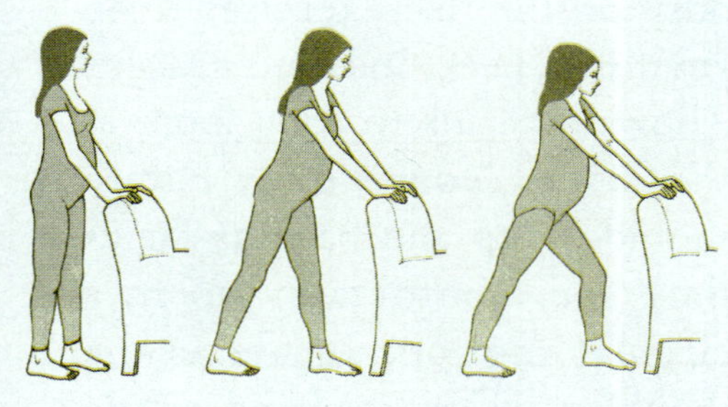

Stand with feet slightly apart and hands on the back of a chair for a secure support. Slide the heel of the right leg back, as far as possible, without letting the heel leave the floor. Then bend the knee of the left leg, lowering yourself slightly as you feel the stretch in the calf muscles of your right leg. Return to original standing position, relax for a few minutes and repeat the exercise with the opposite leg.

The calf stretching exercise is a particularly effective means of relieving leg cramps. If performed regularly, it may also help check cramps.

Stretch the chest muscles

You can do this exercise in a standing or sitting position. Inhale while extending the right arm with the elbow slightly bent above your

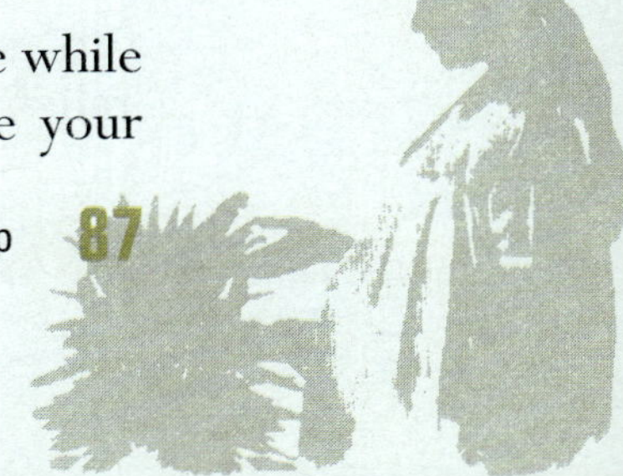

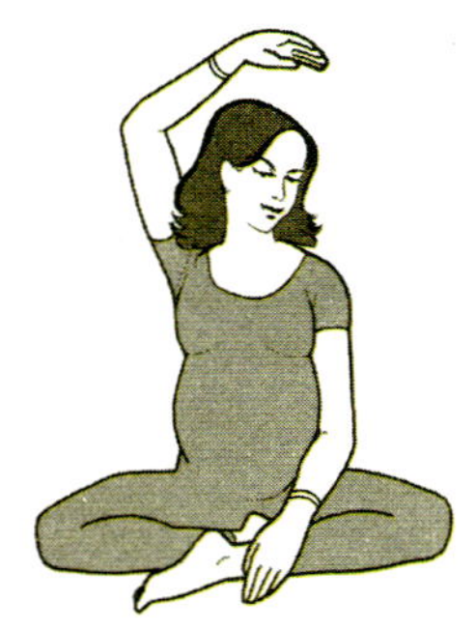

head. Now, straighten the arm and exhale, extending the arm further. Inhale again, return to the starting position and repeat the exercise with the left arm. Repeat the exercise five times with each arm.

The main use of this exercise is in increasing the flexibility and tone of the chest muscles. It can also be used to find relief from shortness of breath.

Rotate the shoulder

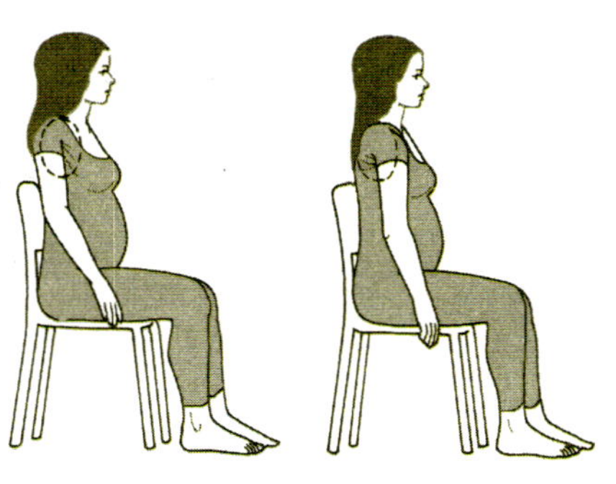

You could take a standing or sitting position for this exercise. Keep your back, neck, and head straight. Allow the arms to hang loose at the sides. Now slowly rotate shoulders up and back as far as they can comfortably go in a circular motion. Inhale as the shoulders are rotated and exhale as the circle is completed and the shoulders have returned to the starting position. Repeat 10 times, relaxing momentarily between each rotation.

This exercise is useful in strengthening the muscles of the upper back and may be used to relieve upper backache and numbness in the arms and fingers.

Relief from discomfort

You can use the different comfort positions and exercises to find relief from some of the common discomforts of pregnancy.

Discomfort	Execise or Position
Swelling of feet, ankles	Leg elevation
Leaking urine while coughing or laughing	Pelvic floor exercises
Heaviness in pelvis	Knee-chest, pelvic floor exercises
Haemorrhoids and swelling around vagina	Knee-chest, pelvic floor exercises
Cramps in thighs, buttocks	Knee-chest
Cramps in legs	Leg elevation, calf stretching
Tired legs	Leg elevation, calf stretching
Varicose veins in legs	Leg elevation, calf stretching
Shortness of breath	Chest muscle stretches, shoulder rotation
Low backache	Pelvic tilt exercise, good posture, squatting position
Upper backache	Shoulder rotation, good posture
Numbness in arms and fingers	Shoulder rotation, lying on side
Spasm in abdominal muscles	Deep abdominal breathing, pelvic tilt

Conscious Relaxation for Easy Childbirth

You must take a few classes under a physiotherapist's supervision to learn conscious relaxation. That will make labour and delivery easy for you. Getting tense during labour is a natural response to the contracting uterus. Tension, however, causes exhaustion, depletes oxygen, lowers the body's tolerance to pain and prolongs labour. That is because adrenaline, the hormone that accompanies the fear-tension-pain syndrome, inhibits the effects of oxytocin. Oxytocin is the natural hormone which causes the uterus to contract. The

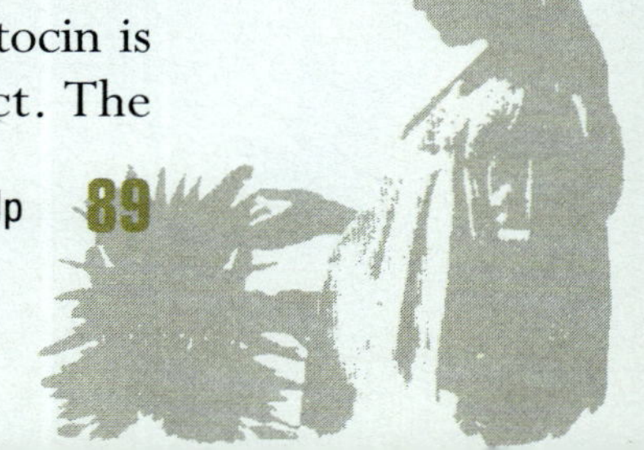

interference of adrenaline with oxytocin therefore makes the contractions of the uterus less effective. This prolongs the process of labour. But if you are able to relax and control at will, childbirth can become much smoother and easier.

Learning to relax at will, however, is rather difficult. It takes an effort to learn and constant practise to master. It requires an active control of mind over body and an excellent concentration. You must develop an active awareness of the state of the muscles, either tense or relaxed and an ability to consciously control that state. You must also learn to identify different muscle groups and be able to consciously release or tense them. You should become so good that it may become a conditioned response. At each contraction, you should spontaneously be able to relax the body completely. This will require constant practice. You must be very regular during the last weeks of pregnancy. Only then would you be able to consciously relax your body during labour. This would permit the muscles of the uterus to work undisturbed, at maximum efficiency and with the least amount of pain.

How to Breathe during Labour

You must also pay attention to breathing exercises. If you breathe in the correct way, pushing the baby out during childbirth becomes that much easier.

Take a complete breath

A complete breath is one in which the chest wall expands and the diaphragm descends to its maximum extent. You should do so periodically during a relaxation phase to fill yourself with oxygen.

1. Breathe in once, as deeply as possible.
2. Hiss or blow the air out slowly, letting your whole body go limp.

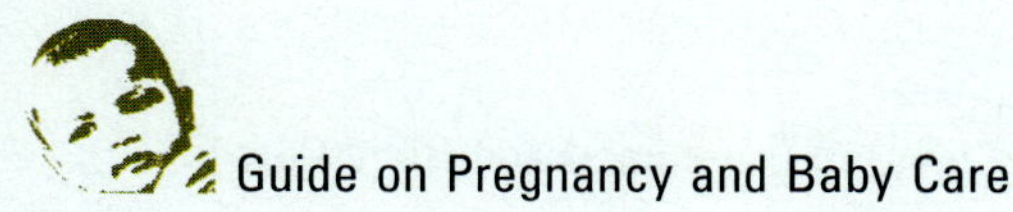

3. Continue breathing quietly, easily and rhythmically.
4. Let yourself go completely loose.
5. Soon your body will begin to feel very heavy and any exertion will be difficult.

Gradually bend an elbow, bringing your hand toward your chin. Notice the effort. Slowly lower your arm to its resting position. Again, you will find yourself working to prevent it from falling too quickly.

Breathe deep during the first stage

1. Pretend that you are having a contraction that lasts 30 to 45 seconds.
2. At the beginning of each contraction take a complete breath and hiss or blow it out.
3. Breathe deeply, slowly and rhythmically throughout the remainder of the contraction.
4. When the contraction has ended, take another complete breath and hiss or blow it out slowly.
5. Breathe normally between contractions.
6. During labour, continue to use this pattern of breathing with contractions as long as it is helpful.

Modify your breathing as contractions get stronger

As labour advances and contractions increase in strength, you often have a desire to keep the diaphragm as still as possible. Yet the uterus continues to need a good supply of oxygen. For this reason you should breathe deeply when the contraction begins and ends, and modify your breathing so that it is quiet and shallow at the peak of each contraction. To practice this, do the following:

1. Pretend that you are having stronger contractions, lasting almost a minute.

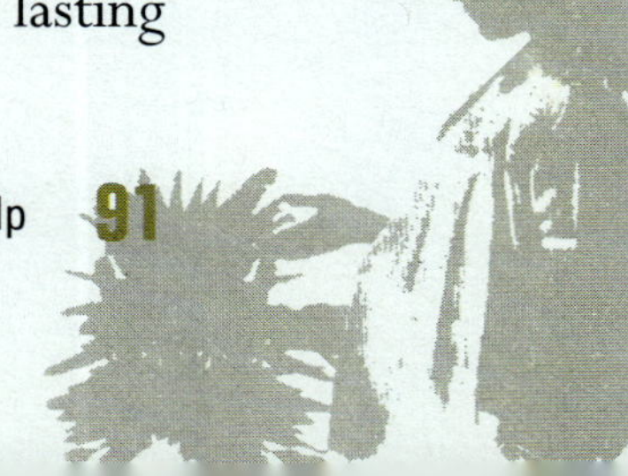

2. Breathe in deeply as the contraction starts. Then slowly hiss or blow out, letting yourself go completely limp.
3. Make each of the next four or five breaths a little shallower than the previous one. You will notice that you are breathing very lightly.
4. Light breathing is quiet and effortless. Find your own comfortable rate and continue for 15 to 45 seconds. If you become dizzy or light headed, your breathing is too vigorous, if you have trouble getting enough air or difficulty maintaining the rhythm, try taking a quick, deep breath and return to light breathing.
5. After the contraction has begun to subside, make each of the next four or five breaths a little deeper than the previous one.
6. End the breath pattern with one complete breath.

Push to help the baby out

During the second stage of labour, you will find that pushing helps in the delivery of the baby. Contractions at this time last 60 to 65 seconds and generally are accompanied by a strong urge to push.

1. Lie on your back with head and shoulders elevated. Pillows may be used for practice at home. In the labour room the head of the bed should be elevated.
2. Bend your knees and separate your legs.
3. Take a deep breath and hiss or blow out.
4. Breathe in as quickly and deeply as you can, then hold your breath. When the actual time comes, this "held" breath will help to fix your diaphragm so that your abdominal wall will make more effective downward pressure on the uterus and the baby, aiding the baby's birth.
5. Draw up your legs against your abdomen in a squatting position, holding your thighs, ankles or feet with your

hands. If a delivery table is used, your feet and legs will be supported in stirrups so that you will not have to hold them and there will be handles on which to pull. Raise your head.

6. During practice, do not actually push. You will be able to do so in labour.
7. Take short breaths when you can no longer hold your breath comfortably as needed. Try to take no more than two or three catch breaths in each 60 to 65 second breath pattern.
   a. Maintain the pushing position.
   b. Exhale, moving your head back.
   c. Take in a quick, deep breath.
   d. Tilt your head forward again and hold your breath.
8. When the contraction is over, relax completely, take a deep breath and sigh it out.

Stop pushing the moment doctor tells you

Your doctor may tell you to stop pushing in the middle of a contraction. If so, start breathing hard immediately. This will make your diaphragm move up and down and physically prevent you from pushing. You could accomplish the same purpose also by blowing forcefully.

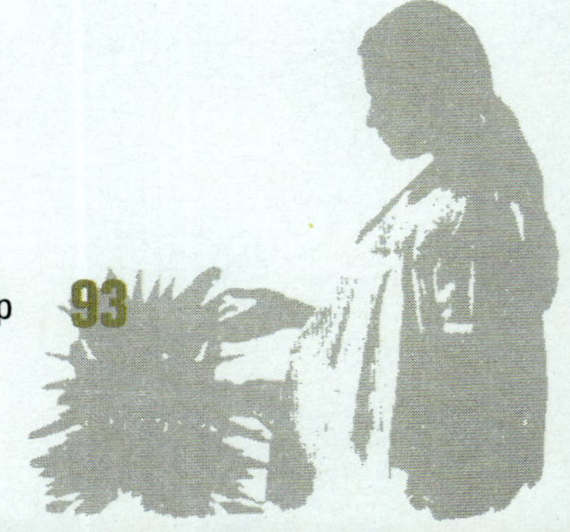

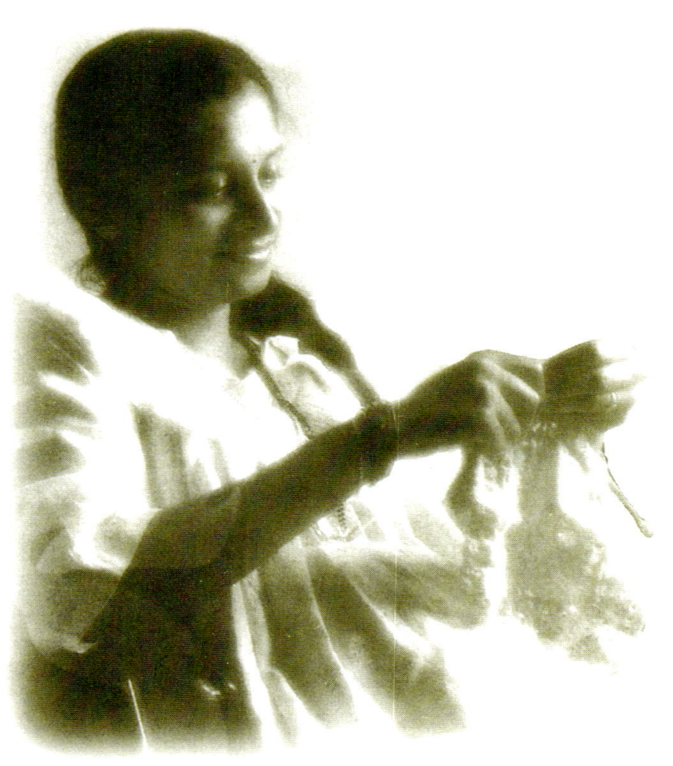

"The sweetest sounds to mortals given
Are heard in Mother, Home and
Heaven"

-W.G. Brown (1812-1906),
English poet.
Mother, Home, Heaven

Sensible Care During Pregnancy

A well-balanced healthy lifestyle is the key to good health at all times. In pregnancy, you just cannot do without this simple wisdom. You may continue to work right till the baby is born, but strike a balance between work and rest. Too vigorous exercise and strenuous sports are out, but walking, simple exercises and regular sports are in. You can feel and act normal, but never lose the shelter of sensible care.

At Work

Most workingwomen want to carry on working while they are pregnant, until they take maternity leave. Mothers at home with children have no choice but to work right through to the end of pregnancy. Sometimes working can be quite difficult, especially if you feel sick and tired in the early months. To keep yourself going, and to care for your baby, just follow some simple sensible advice:

- Eat properly. Try to have something to eat before you start work in the morning. If you feel sick, take a cereal, corn flakes and milk or toast. If you really cannot eat early, have a snack at ten, when you feel less sick. Include some fresh fruit in your lunch. If you cannot get fruit where you work, take it with you from home.
- Try to have a quiet sit down after lunch, even it is only for

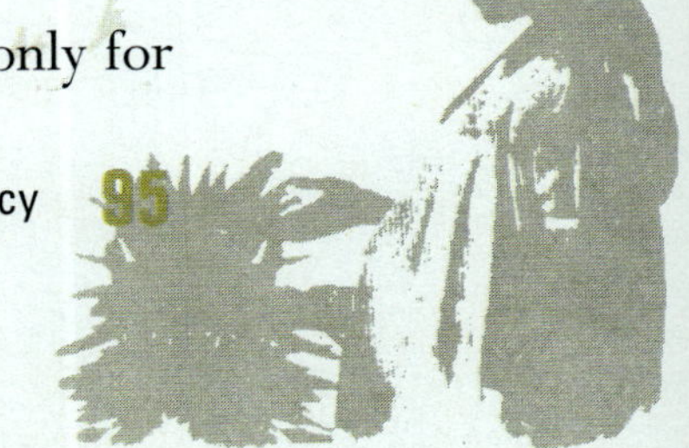

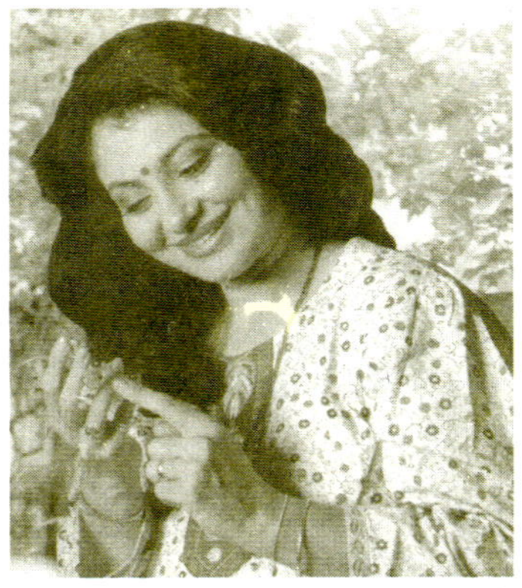

a short time. Just put your feet up (if the office environment permits) on a stool, rest your head on the table and relax. Take another breather in the evening. And if daytime resting is out of the question, at least make sure you get good rest in bed at night. If travelling in the rush hour gets very difficult for you, talk to your employer about the possibility of working slightly different hours for while.

- If you already have children, try to find someone who will look after them for you for at least an hour or so every now and then. A break will be good for you and for them. If you live as a nuclear family, ask a close relative such as your mother, mother-in-law or sister to shift in and help.
- Take a domestic help or ask your spouse to help with the housework. Even if you can get a part-time maid, it would make a big difference. She could complete some of the more exacting housework and you can take some time out.
- Remember that you have a right to take time off work to go for antenatal care without losing pay (see page 223), and the right to return to your job after you have had your baby.

If you work with chemicals or lead or are exposed to radiation, or if the work you do is very tiring, then it could be risky to go on working while you're pregnant. Check on any risks that you think there may be. If there is a risk, you can ask to be moved to another, safer job.

Exercise, sports and rest

When you are pregnant you need some rest and some exercise just as you normally do. You may find that you get tired more easily, especially in the early months and later in your pregnancy. If you do feel tired, take rest. Go to bed earlier at night or if it is possible have a rest in the middle of the day. You may at least be able to do this at weekends. If you would rather not rest in bed, relax by having a quiet hour or so sitting down with your feet up.

But if you have been sitting all day, then it is good to get moving. Do whatever feels right and makes you feel good. Do not make yourself get exhausted, but do not let yourself get sluggish either. Remember, if you are feeling tense after a day's work, exercise can be relaxing. Take a walk daily. A regular 20-30 minute walk keeps both your body and mind in order, improves circulation in the legs and tones you up.

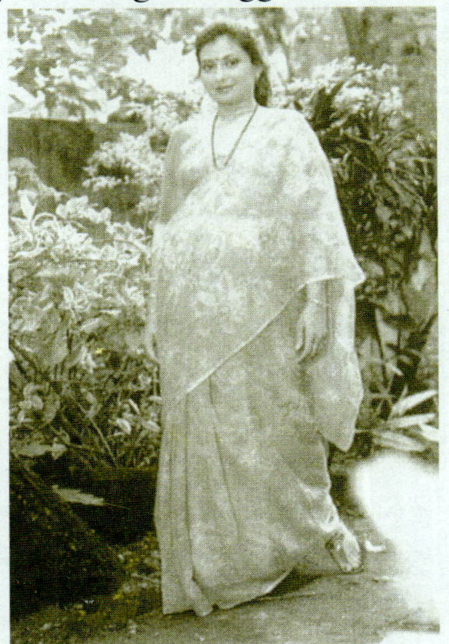

For those who enjoy swimming, a game of badminton or table tennis, there is certainly no reason why you should not go on doing so. Play any sensible sport you wish, as long as you feel comfortable.

Clothing and footwear

It is best to wear loose fitting clothes. Gowns and loose flowing robes are probably the best. But if you feel like, you can even pick designer clothes, which suit your size and requirement and go with your personality. Tight clothes are not suitable. Wearing them can worsen indigestion and heartburn because they would promote reflux of acid. They also increase the risk of fungal infection in the vagina.

A word about footwear—avoid the use of high-heeled shoes. They can strain the back and throw you off balance. This is particularly so when the pregnancy enters an advanced state. You must also take care to avoid footwear that may predispose you to tripping, slipping and falling.

Travel

You can travel as much as you wish, provided this can be carried out in a leisurely manner without any undue stress or strain. There is no restriction on flying or travelling by train. However, it is wise to consider the possible implications of long journeys during the later months of pregnancy. Nearer term, it is best to stay close to home, unless you wish to risk childbirth somewhere on the way.

Sex

There is no reason why you should discontinue sex in normal pregnancy. Having sex does not harm the baby because the penis cannot penetrate beyond the vagina. The muscles of the cervix and a plug of mucus formed in pregnancy seal off the womb completely.

However, if you have had a previous miscarriage you may decide not to have an intercourse in the first three or four months of pregnancy. It is probably safer that way. If at any time you experience slight bleeding, vaginal or abdominal pain, it is best to abstain and take complete rest.

Later in pregnancy, an orgasm can set off contractions. These are the sort of contractions that you will notice from time to time right through the second half of pregnancy. You will feel the muscles of your womb go hard. If this is uncomfortable after an intercourse, just lie quietly until the contractions pass.

While sex is safe for most couples in pregnancy, you may need to make some adjustments. For instance, you would probably need to try different positions. The man-on-top can become rather uncomfortable, not just because of the baby, but because of tender breasts as well. It can also be uncomfortable for the woman if the man's penis penetrates too deeply. So it may be better to lie on your sides, either facing, or with the man behind or opt for the woman-on-top position.

It is probably best to avoid intercourse during the last six weeks because it can possibly allow ingress to unfriendly bacteria, thus opening you to infection during the post childbirth period.

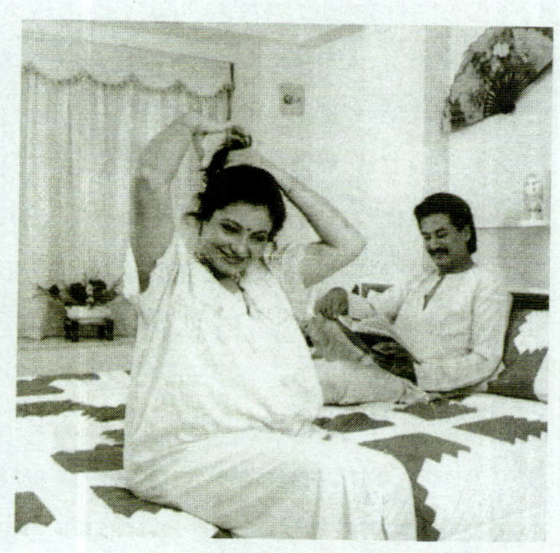

In any case, some couples simply feel that they do not want to have intercourse during pregnancy and find other ways of making love and being loved. If you feel that way, it is perfectly all right.

Smoking, Alcohol and Medicines

Smoking

Call it quits today, because the dangers smoking poses to pregnancy are simply too many. It harms your own health and that of your baby, by holding back its growth. You run a greater risk of complications when your baby is born. There is a higher risk that your baby will be premature and underweight. Babies of women who smoke are on average 200 g lighter than they should be.

The nicotine, that you inhale, passes into your baby's bloodstream. Among other things, this makes your baby's heart beat too fast. The carbon monoxide from the cigarette also passes into your bloodstream. This means that the blood carries less oxygen. The baby also therefore gets less oxygen and cannot grow well.

Alcohol

Keep alcohol to the minimum and certainly not more than 30-60 ml per day. It is known that heavy drinking during pregnancy can affect the development of the baby adversely, especially during the early weeks. More recently, some evidence has suggested that even moderate or light drinking can affect the baby in the same way though less severely.

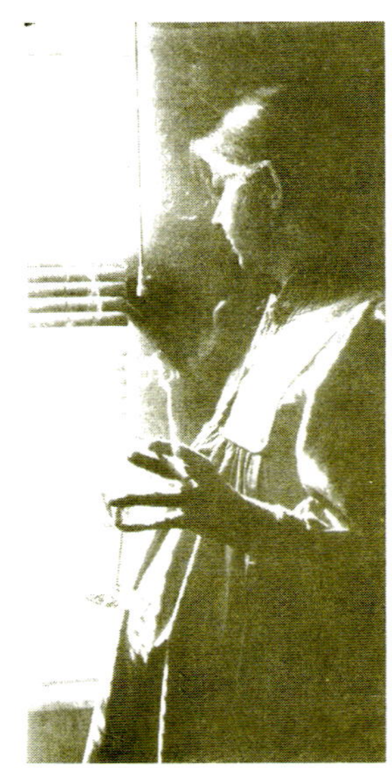

Remember, from conception onwards, the less you drink, the better are your chances of a successful pregnancy and a healthy baby. It is true that if you limit yourself to just an occasional drink, the risk to your baby will be very small. But if you cut out alcohol completely, you cut out this risk completely. Often it is, when you are with other people who are drinking that it is hardest to resist alcohol. Try find a non-alcoholic drink you like and stick to that.

Pills and Medicines

Do tell the doctor or dentist that you are pregnant before they prescribe any medicine. Even medicines that you can buy over-the-counter may not be safe and these include those of the alternative systems. If you are on a regular medication, discuss its safety with the doctor. Medication should never be taken in pregnancy without good reason particularly in the first three months. The doctor should be sure about the need for medication and the choice of medicines must be based on an evidence of large-scale studies rather than individual fancy. The safety of dosage and duration of therapy should also be fully taken note of. This is particularly so when considering the use of a new drug. A tragic example was the use of thalidomide, a hypnotic drug, the use of which has been associated with multiple foetal malformations. But a number of other medications are also known to have detrimental effects and a list is presented below.

Medicines which can cause abnormalities in your baby

Medicine	Abnormality
Androgens/ Progestagens	Masculinisation of female foetus
Anti thyroid drugs	Goitre
Chloroquine (prolonged excessive use)	Inner ear (vestibular) damage
Chlorpropamide (anti diabetic pill)	Intrauterine death
Glucocorticoids (steroids)	Retardation of baby's intrauterine growth
Methotrexate (anti metabolite)	Multiple abnormalities
Oestrogens	Cancer of vagina
Anti epilepsy drugs	Hare lip/palate, congenital heart disease, finger abnormalities
Warfarin (blood thinning agent)	Defect in bones
Operating room environment	Abortion, baby's death, probably birth defects
Hormonal pregnancy tests	Developmental malformations
Tetracyclines	Tooth discoloration, impaired bone growth
Thiazides (water pills)	Reduction in number of platelets
Thalidomide (hypnotic)	Limb defects and deformities

Medicines which may be associated with abnormalities in babies

Medicine	Abnormality
Amphetamines (mood elevator)	Defects of the heart absence of bile passages
Antimetabolite drugs	Abnormalities of the eye
Phenobarbitone and Phenytoin	Reduced head circumference, chromosome abnormalities
Phenytoin (anti epileptic)	Abnormalities of the skeleton
Tolbutamide (anti diabetic)	Multiple abnormalities
Sulphonamides (anti microbial)	Liver necrosis, congenital cataracts
LSD (recreational drug)	Chromosome abnormalities
Tetracyclines	Congenital cataracts
Progestagens (hormones)	Hypospadias, multiple congenital abnormalities
Tricyclic anti depressants	Limb defects

Protection From Radiation

Stay away from all radiation sources such as x-ray examination rooms, radiation treatment rooms and industries which employ radiation sources. Radiation during pregnancy can damage the baby and this risk can be eased by following a rule which states that a woman should be X-rayed only within the first 10 days of her menstrual cycle unless the X-ray is required for an urgent reason. The application of this rule limits the possibility of a fertilised egg receiving X-ray radiation. If your doctor however feels that an X-ray examination is absolutely essential for you, you must take the examination. Just request the radiographer to give you suitable protection. If the X-ray is of some other part, a lead apron can be placed on the abdomen.

You must also avoid standing in an X-ray examination room for a relative or friend. If you have an older child who needs to be examined, your spouse can attend on the child.

The Power of Logic

Never bother about the dozens of illogical, unscientific restrictions well-meaning grandmas and older women like to impose on mothers- and fathers-to-be. For instance, tying any knots, knitting, hanging out clothes on the washline is taboo. That is completely irrational and absurd, and rather impractical if you live as a nuclear family.

Likewise, there is so much hullabaloo about a solar or lunar eclipse, were it to occur during your pregnancy. You will be told to lie in a bed in a closed room and not to stir out of it as long as the eclipse lasts. You may also be offered weighty and seemingly scientific explanations for this belief. But all that talk of ultraviolet rays penetrating through the mother, and in turn harming the baby, is plain and simple bunkum. Do not be swayed by it or feel anxious.

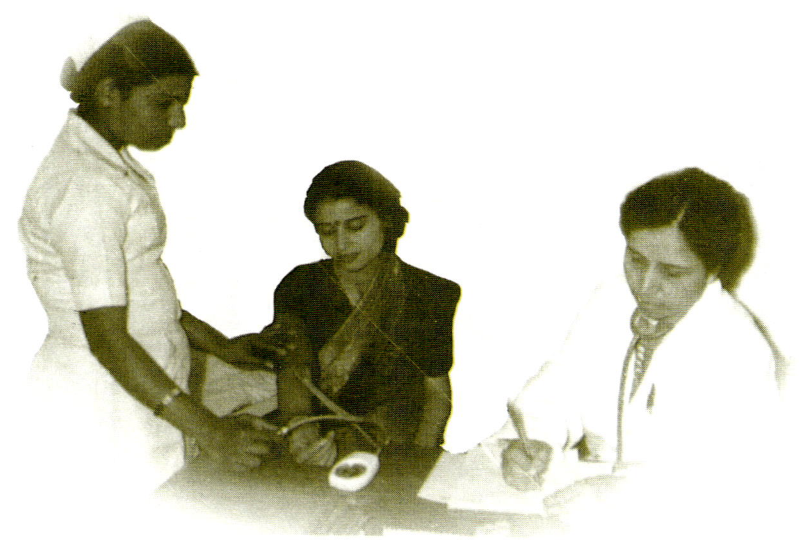

"The aim of antenatal care during pregnancy is to preserve its naturalness, and the ideal result . . . a healthy mother in possession of a healthy child."

– Sir Eardley Holland,
British obstetrician

All About Doctors and Tests

The basis of sound antenatal care is simply regular sensible medical attention. A natural process, pregnancy and childbirth do not brook much interference. The regular check-ups at the antenatal clinic or with your own doctor are just to make sure that both you and the baby are fit and well, to check that the baby is developing properly and as far as possible to prevent anything going wrong, either during your pregnancy or when you go into labour.

Choice of Doctor

A regular check-up is most important from the moment you believe that you may be pregnant and till you have made a full recovery from the rigours of childbirth, hence there is a need to find a good doctor.

The obstetrician must be well experienced and readily available at the time of your need. There is no point in seeking an appointment with a very prominent obstetrician, only to be told that she is not available when you are in need.

All obstetricians are usually closely associated with certain hospitals or nursing homes, where they would take you in at the time of childbirth. Such a hospital has to be well geared to cope with any emergency that may arise. There is absolutely no doubt that many small centres are ill equipped to cope with some of the serious complications that can arise suddenly and without warning. This means there is a high risk to the mother and the infant at the time of birth. Do not take such a risk.

Choice of Hospital

The place should be clean and equipped with facilities to tide over any sudden emergency. Shifting the mother at the eleventh hour just because this or that facility does not exist can be extremely risky. There is often, little or no time for that.

Courteous and attentive nursing staff, clean environment, spotless bed sheets, well prepared food all reflect on the institution, but it is equally important to look at the practical side of things. If the hospital, no matter how good it is, happens to be located many miles from where you live and is difficult to access, then it may not be the most convenient place after all. Of course, with confinement number one, there is usually plenty of warning time.

Also, check out the charges beforehand, without feeling shy or ashamed. Asking for the full cost may be better, as this way you exclude the possibility of hidden costs. You may also decide on a public healthcare facility to restrict the expenses. Most public hospitals and clinics in India offer antenatal service for free, although there may be some nominal charge for extended facilities and bed. Some of the larger hospitals many ask you to book in advance, in the first three months of your being pregnant.

Calculating Baby's Arrival Date

When the pregnancy is confirmed, most mothers wish to know, "When will the baby be born?" This is a reasonable query and one can very easily work out the answer for oneself. The actual duration of pregnancy is 266 days, on an average. This is the number of days from the moment conception occurs, to the moment the baby is born. However, for the point of convenience, doctors customarily measure dates, not from the time of conception, but from the first day of the last menstrual cycle. This, in a woman with a normal 26- to 32-day cycle, is 280 days.

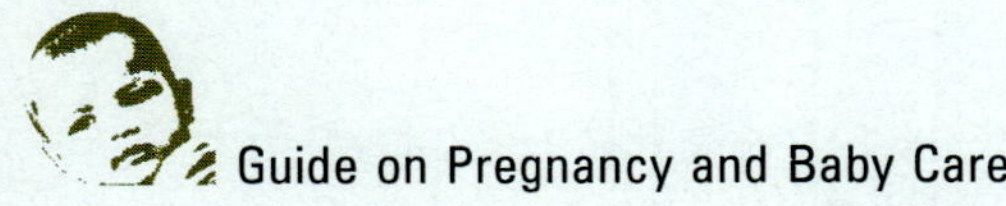

The abbreviation LMP is widely used by doctors to refer to this important date and it stands for the last menstrual period. From this date, the time of the baby's arrival can be readily calculated. This is referred to as the, "estimated date of delivery," or EDD for short.

To avoid the time-consuming job of sitting down and adding 280 days to the LMP, charts have been worked out which clearly indicate this. The top line gives the LMP for each day of the year. Directly underneath is given the EDD, corresponding to each date. This chart gives you the near date for delivery. The bookmark tagged to this book offers this chart. Do use it!

Use Mental Arithmetic

There is another simple method. Simply, add seven days to the LMP and count back three months. That gives a fairly accurate date and this is projected ahead. For example, let's say the LMP was September 13. September 13 + 7 days = September 20, less three months = June 20. The EDD will then be June 20 the following year.

It is as simple as that and remarkably accurate.

Other Methods

There are various other methods of determining the baby's birth date.

Ultrasound

If all is normal, the ultrasound doctor's observations can be taken as a very good estimate. But if the baby is not growing according to his gestational age, the EDD given by the sonologist may well be fallacious.

The date of quickening

The "time of quickening" can also be used as a rough guide. This is when movements are first felt. But as this can vary between the 16th and 24th week, it is of limited use. As a rough estimate, the EDD can be taken to be five months from the date the baby first begins to show active movements.

The height of the uterus

As time progresses, the doctor usually measures the height of the fundus on each visit. This means that she presses her hand into the abdomen to determine the upper extent of the growing womb. The womb enlarges at a fairly constant rate, and the height, as it is called, usually coincides with the number of weeks of development of the baby. At 12 weeks the fundus is just starting to edge above the symphysis, the front part of the bony pelvis. By 16 weeks, it has risen to midway between the symphysis and the navel. It has reached 22-24 weeks when it rises to the level of the navel. About the 36th week the uterus attains its greatest height in the abdomen, extending nearly to the lower tip of the breastbone and the abdominal girth may reach 36 inches. During

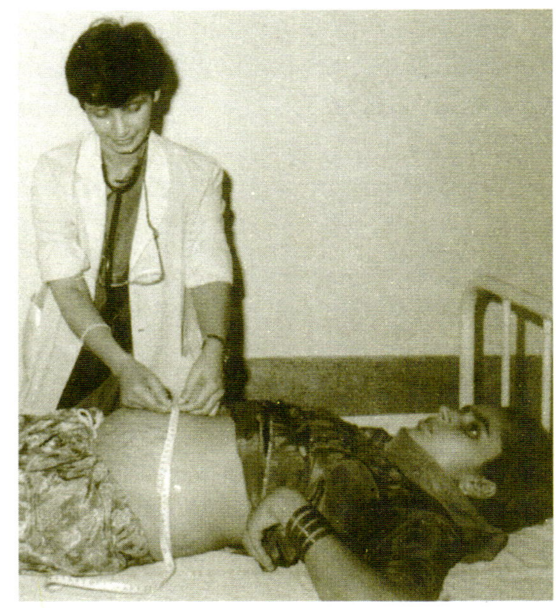

the last fortnight of pregnancy, it usually sinks by about an inch. This fundal height is a good guide for the doctor. If the fundus is rising too rapidly, or if it is not rising at the normally anticipated rate, it means that all is not well and an investigation may be required as to the reason.

Objectives of Obstetric Care

The importance and significance of regular antenatal visits to the doctor cannot be overstressed. It is essential that attendance be made as early as is practical. There is no knowing at the start if you are destined to be one of those special "at risk" persons.

There are three major aims for following through with adequate antenatal care. These are:

(1) To make sure that the mother reaches the end of pregnancy healthy or maybe even healthier than what she was.

(2) To detect any physical or psychological defect in the mother as early as possible and correct this promptly.

(3) To deliver a normal healthy baby.

The Antenatal Care Routine

For women with normal pregnancy, it is best that until the 24th week they meet with their doctor every four weeks. After this, fortnightly visits should take place until the 36th week. Visits then become weekly occurrences until the baby is born.

In the event of any problem visits will be more frequent. This will be left to the doctor to tell you when she expects you to return for a subsequent check.

Do not go against your doctor's advice. Do not think you are somebody, who can be excluded from the need of a proper regular medical examination.

First Visit

Most women go to an antenatal clinic for the first time between the eighth 12th weeks of pregnancy. The earlier you go the better. If there is anything wrong, however slight, then it is best to find out early so that the problem can be dealt with. This also allows the doctor to record your baseline vital parameters which cannot be obtained when the pregnancy has advanced.

Your first visit to the clinic is likely to be your longest, where you will be asked a lot of questions:

I. History of the present pregnancy. The doctor will check your LMP. She will ask all the details in an effort to pinpoint whether you are or are not pregnant. In many cases it is quite clear and fairly obvious that you are pregnant.

II. History of previous pregnancies. The doctor will be interested to know about previous pregnancies, whether they proceeded to full term or ended up as miscarriages or abortions. She will want to know about any special difficulties that occurred during the pregnancy or afterwards. Also, if the babies were normal, and the approximate duration of each labour. All this will assist her when it comes to assessing the present case. She may also question you about blood transfusions.

III. History of past illnesses. As certain diseases may be of significance, she will query you on past and present illnesses. Any birth or acquired defects in the heart, epilepsy, diabetes and kidney disorders may be very important.

IV. Physical examination. The doctor will then carry out a full physical examination. Each system is checked. The heart, lungs and abdomen are examined, as well as all other areas.

The breasts and nipples are checked. The doctor will be keen to know your average weight before you became pregnant. She will check your weight and height and blood pressure. In fact, a regular blood pressure reading forms one of the most important checks thereafter. It is essential for the doctor to have a baseline reading with which she can compare subsequent readings.

V. Internal examination. The doctor may decide to carry out an internal examination at this stage. For this, she would ask you to empty your bladder. She may insert an instrument called a speculum into the vagina. This will give her an excellent view of the vaginal passage and the cervix. She will inspect each part thoroughly. If there are discharges, she will probably take a specimen for testing. A cervical smear test will probably be done and sent to the pathological laboratory for examination. This is followed by a manual examination, when she would feel the womb with her fingers and record its size and position. If she notices any abnormalities, their detection now could play an important part later.

VI. Laboratory tests. The doctor will arrange for certain important tests to be carried out. These will usually include various blood tests.

(i) A haemoglobin estimation is performed. This indicates the quality of the blood. If reduced, it is diagnostic of anaemia and the doctor may give treatment.

(ii) The blood group must be known, for this could be vital later on in the event of abnormal bleeding. It is called the "ABO" grouping. In addition, the Rh (or Rhesus) factor must be known. This is also very important for all women, but especially in the cases of mothers pregnant for the first time. This is partly for the records, in case a transfusion should ever be needed. It is also to find mothers whose blood group is rhesus negative. This is not a worry for a first baby. But all rhesus negative mothers who are wedded to rhesus positive men are given an injection after the birth of their first baby to protect their next baby.

(iii) The VDRL and the HIV tests are performed to check against venereal disease.

(iv) A simple urine test (urinalysis) is carried out. This is mainly done to check for albumin and sugar, and to rule out infection. Sometimes a special culture of the urine may also be asked for if the doctor has any suspicion that infection is present in the urinary tract.

(v) If there is any doubt about pregnancy, the pregnancy test may be carried out as well. This is the check for HCG, which has already been explained (see page 50).

Subsequent Visits

An appointment will be made for your next visit. It shall be in four weeks' time. Subsequent visits will be shorter than the initial one. They will chiefly entail a check on the blood pressure, a urine check and weight gain. The mother-to-be can tell her doctor of any abnormality that she has noted.

After the 28th week, examinations tend to be more comprehensive. The doctor will carry out an abdominal check as well as the foregoing procedures. She will assess the height of the fundus and this an indication of the rate at which the baby is growing. She will also check the position of the baby as it lies in the womb.

She can readily work out where each part of the body is, where the head is located, the back and breech. She will listen for the foetal heart sounds and check on its degree of activity. All these are important features and variations from the normal may need to be followed with other investigations.

Vaccinations

It would be in your and your baby's interest to be protected against tetanus. If you have taken the immunisation in the past, you just take a booster of the tetanus toxoid. That would cover you for the next five years. If you have not been immunised, take two shots of the tetanus toxoid, first at 16-20 weeks, the second at 20-25 weeks.

Why Go For These Checks

Some mothers begin to think that these tests are just a routine and possibly avoidable. But that is not correct. Each test is carried out for its merit. It is to make certain that the mother and the developing foetus are safe and there is no risk to them. Tests are never done haphazardly and just for something to do. Let us consider what they are good for.

The weight measurements are important because if the mother-to-be were to gain more than 0.5 kg a week, the doctor stands warned; there is an increased risk of toxaemia, one of the serious complications of pregnancy. Likewise, blood pressure readings are very important. A reading of 140/90 points is taken as the upper limit of normal. If pressure readings touch or cross these figures, it is a cause for concern and action. Urine tests check albumin, which is a protein substance. Once more, it can be a warning signal that serious medical complications may be starting, and action is imperative at once.

Blood checks have considerable significance as well. The haemoglobin level gives a clear, accurate assessment of the mother's blood quality. This is done at the start. If it shows a reduced level, special treatment may be prescribed to bring it up to the normal level. A recheck is then required. So, reassessments may take place occasionally, depending on what the doctor considers necessary.

From time to time, the doctor may consider other tests are needed. Go with her advice. Most doctors would want you to go for the ultrasound test, and more than one may be necessary.

Special tests

Using special tests, it is now possible to find out a great deal about the baby while it is still in the womb. Certain tests in the first half of pregnancy, for example, can detect serious abnormalities so that, if the parents wish it, the pregnancy can be ended.

The Ultrasound Test

Ultrasound is a completely safe and painless test which uses high frequency sound waves to present a true picture of your baby. You lie on your back under the scanner, a jelly is applied on your lower abdomen and a small device called transducer is passed backwards and forwards over your skin. The high intensity sound waves beamed by the transducer reach the inner organs. The echo is reflected back and this is picked by the transducer to create live pictures on a monitor screen which is much like a TV. It can be most exciting to see a picture of your baby before birth.

This examination can be done at any stage of pregnancy. The first is usually done at about 16 or 17 weeks to check for any congenital malformations. At this stage, your bladder should be nearly full when you go for the scan. A second scan may be carried out at 32 to 36 weeks of pregnancy to confirm that the baby is growing well, but it is not necessary in the absence of any risk markers.

Most hospitals perform at least one ultrasound scan during a pregnancy. This is for several reasons. A scan can give quite an accurate idea of the baby's age and when it will be born, which helps if you are unsure about the date of your last period. It shows the placenta, the adequacy or not of amniotic fluid and the presentation of the baby. A scan can also help detect abnormalities, particularly of the baby's head or spine. It can also help to detect twins or multiple pregnancies. It is also a most useful tool in the following situations:

- Locating the cause of bleeding or abdominal pain during early pregnancy

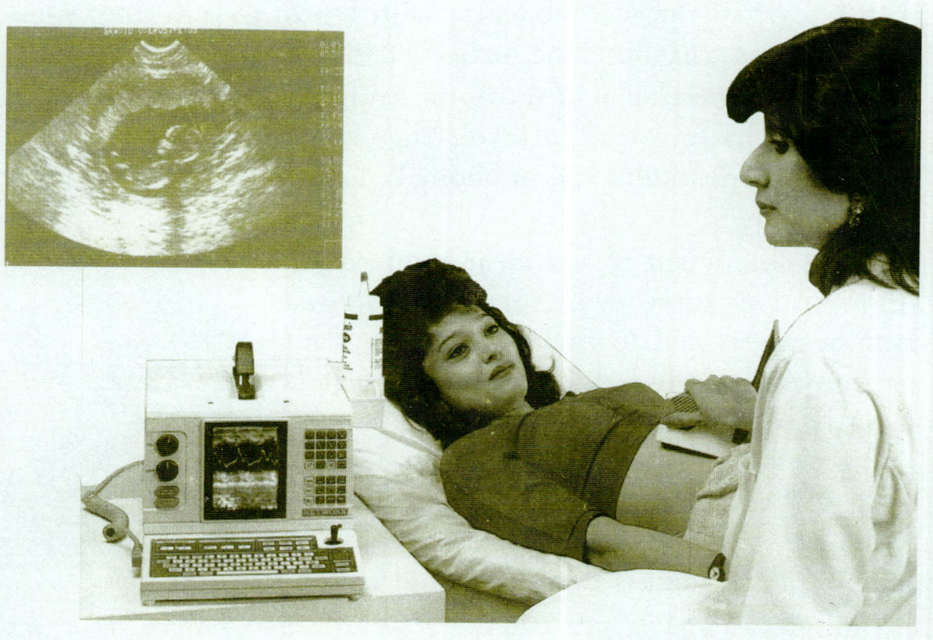

- To check for baby's size and liquor volume when the uterus is small or large for dates
- For a detailed examination of the baby when the risk of congenital anomaly is high or an amniocentesis or chorionic villi sampling is to be done
- Looking for foetal defects when serum AFP levels are found to be high
- Monitoring foetal growth in high-risk pregnancies
- For checking out the cause of baby's distress

Amniocentesis

This test is performed very occasionally. It is recommended in the following situations:

- For older mothers (over 35 years) who run a higher risk of having a baby with Down's syndrome,
- When there is someone with Down's syndrome, spina bifida, haemophilia or muscular dystrophy in the family,
- For women whose blood sample has shown a raised alpha-fetoprotein level, suggesting the possibility of an anomaly in the baby.

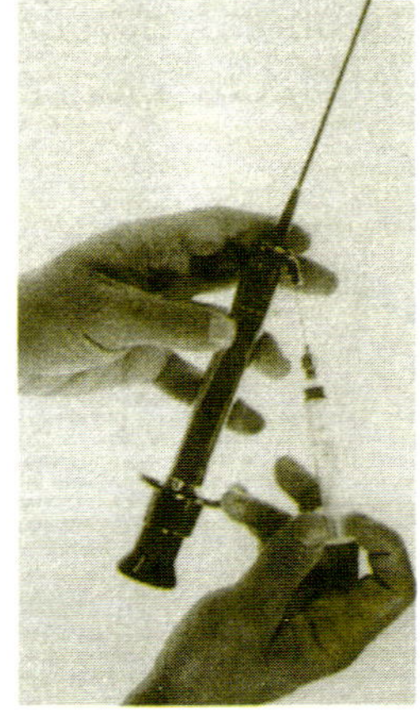

It is important to get clear information on why exactly you are having an amniocentesis and to find out all you want to know about it beforehand. The test is usually done around 16-18 weeks of pregnancy. A needle is pushed through the wall of the abdomen into the amniotic fluid which surrounds the baby in the womb. A sample of the fluid is drawn out and tested.

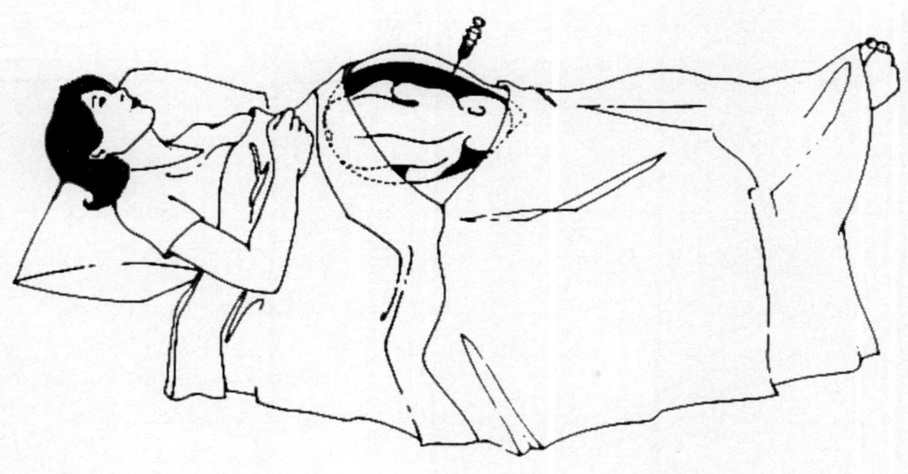

The technique of aminocentesis

The results of the test are known in a few days, but if the test has been done to exclude Down's syndrome, it is more complicated and takes a few weeks. The genetic test also reveals the baby's sex. If there is haemophilia or muscular dystrophy in your family, it's important to know the baby's sex. If it is a boy, he may inherit the disease.

An ultrasound scan is always done before an amniocentesis to check the position of the baby and placenta so that the needle damages neither. All the same, there is a slight risk that the amniocentesis will cause a miscarriage. Just over 1 in 100 tests result in the loss of the baby. In deciding whether or not to go ahead with an amniocentesis, you need to balance this risk against what would be the value or benefit of the test for you.

Check If You Are A High Risk Mother

Some situations carry a high risk for the mother and the baby. Here is an account of such markers and their adverse fall-outs.

Marker	Risk(s)
Teenage pregnancy	Baby being born premature, being of low birth weight, dying soon after or within the first year of birth.
Maternal age over 35 years	Increase risk of Down's syndrome.
Maternal age over 40 years	As above; also the risk of toxaemia, pre-term and precipitate labour and baby presenting to the birth canal in the wrong way. Increased risk to mother and baby.
Smoking (10 or more cigarettes a day)	Increased risk of baby developing poorly and of being born before term.
Alcohol (>60 ml alcohol daily)	Mental retardation in the baby, premature delivery leading to increased risk to mother and baby.
Drug abuse	Increased risk of miscarriage, poor growth of the baby, premature delivery, risk of hepatitis and HIV infection.
Inheritable diseases: Personal or family history of genetic disorders such as haemoglobin disorders, heart defects, cleft lip and palate, schizophrenia and birth malformations in mother, father, family or previous child.	Risk of the same defect in the baby. The risk varies with the nature of inheritance of a particular defect.

Diabetes in first-degree relatives of the pregnant mother	Higher risk of diabetes in pregnancy.
Past history of developing a clot	Risk of recurrence.
Mismatch of blood groups between the husband and wife; wife being Rh negative	Intra uterine death of the baby, baby being born with jaundice and anaemia.
Multiple pregnancy	Higher risk of miscarriage, premature delivery, toxaemia, anaemia and vaginal bleeding.
Previous Caesarean Section	Dehiscence of scar.
Past history of premature placental separation	Risk of recurrence and severe blood loss, loss of baby.
Past history of severe (third degree) tear in the perineum at the time of childbirth	Risk of a damage to anal sphincter.
Infertility and (or) recurrent misc-carriage in the past	Miscarriage, multiple pregnancies, ectopic pregnancy.
Psychological factors:	
Recent divorce, separation or major family upset	Premature delivery.
Past history of depressive or some other serious psychiatric illness	Psychological distress may worsen during pregnancy or after childbirth.

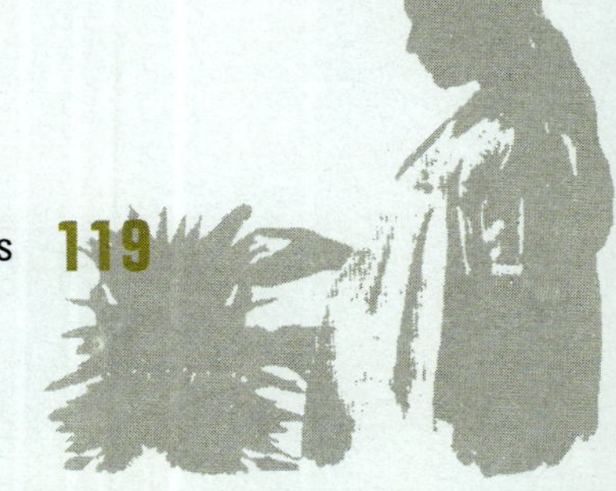

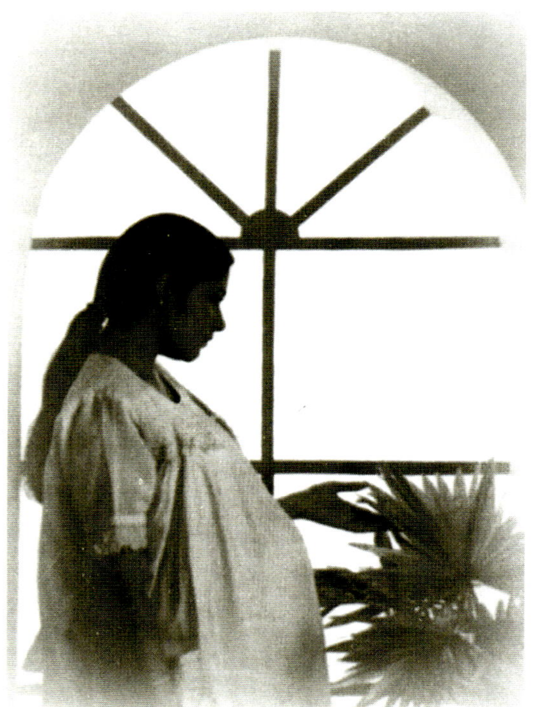

"Man needs difficulties; they are necessary for health."

-Carl Jung (1875-1961), Swiss psychiatrist.
The Transcendent Function

Common Problems During Pregnancy

Minor problems are common during pregnancy. Almost all pregnant mothers endure them. But the key is not to let these annoyances get the better of you. Overcoming them is easy provided you know what is causing them and what to do about them. You should also recognise the signs when a minor problem needs expert attention. If, at any time in your pregnancy, for any reason, you feel worried about something, the best course is to consult your doctor.

Nausea and morning sickness

Nausea in the early weeks of pregnancy is a common occurrence. It affects eight in 10 pregnant women. But fortunately, less than 40 per cent mothers complain of vomiting. The symptoms can begin as early as in the fourth week, but generally disappear by the 12th to 14th week. However, some mothers are not that lucky and continue to suffer right up to the 20th week.

The intensity and pattern of symptoms varies in each person. While some simply feel overcome with nausea, others cannot digest anything and begin to throw up. Some feel the symptoms in the mornings, some at other times, some all day long. The exact mechanism of this symptom is not clearly known but the hormonal changes that occur during early pregnancy definitely play a major role.

What to do

To find relief, try the following suggestions:

- Eat small meals within short gaps, instead of the usual three meals a day. Many mothers feel well with this small change in routine.
- If you feel worst first thing in the morning, eat a dry toast or plain biscuit before you get up.
- Avoid foods and smells that make you feel worse. If you are cooking for the family, choose menus that will suit you as well as them. For yourself, eat foods that make you feel better and are equally good for health.
- Try cold foods because they have less aroma than hot foods—the sense of smell is very acute during pregnancy.
- Wear comfortable clothes. Tightly bound clothing around the waist can make you feel worse.
- Distract yourself as much as you can—often nausea worsens the more you think about it.
- Severe vomiting is rare. If it is persists, you run the risk of dehydration and electrolyte imbalance. Contact the doctor. If necessary, she can arrange for a short stay in hospital to correct the fluid imbalance. It may also be necessary to exclude a urinary tract infection.
- If you develop nausea towards the end of pregnancy, visit your doctor for blood pressure and urine check-up.

Indigestion and heartburn

During pregnancy many women discover that foods they normally enjoy now give them indigestion. One obvious solution is to avoid foods that cause the trouble. But make sure that your diet is still well balanced. In general, try eating smaller meals more often, and sit straight while eating. This takes pressure off your stomach.

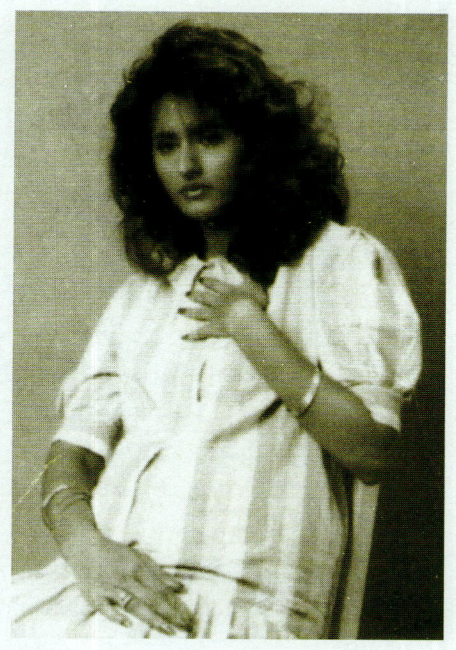

Heartburn is more than just indigestion. It is a strong, burning pain in the chest caused by the abnormal relaxation of the valve between your stomach and the food pipe. This allows the acid in the stomach to pass into the food pipe. Over 50 per cent of all pregnant women suffer from heartburn. The reasons are twofold: one, the growing baby pushes the stomach upwards, and two, the hormone of pregnancy (progesterone) relaxes the valve.

Heartburn is often brought on by large meals or lying flat. It, therefore, makes sense to try and break you meal into smaller, more manageable portions. You must also avoid lying flat or bending down after partaking a meal. Sit in a comfortable upright position, so that the food can progress to the small intestine. Also sleep well propped up, with the head of the bed raised. Drinking milk can also help. Keep a glass of milk by your side in case you wake with heartburn in the night. You may also try simple antacid mixtures or tablets such as magnesium trisilicate. Avoid the regular heartburn tablets such as cimetidine, ranitidine and famotidine which are absorbed into the bloodstream and are therefore, not very safe.

Dizziness

Pregnant women often feel faint. Bouts of dizziness can occur if you stand still after walking briskly or if you get up from a low chair or get out of bed in a hurry. They can also occur when you are lying on your back.

What to do

If you feel dizzy while standing, sit down quickly and wait for the spell to pass. If you are lying on your back, turn onto your left side. This particularly applies when the pregnancy is in the later stages. Turning to one side takes the pressure off the big vein (inferior vena cava) and produces immediate relief by increasing blood circulation.

Headaches

Headaches are a common complaint with some pregnant women. This again is because of the hormones.

What to do

Avoid hot, stuffy surroundings. Rest and relax. Drink plenty of liquids. Bathe regularly and enjoy the coolness of water in any form. If the headache persists, you can take an ordinary paracetamol tablet, but not aspirin. Paracetamol is safe and does not harm the baby.

If the headaches are frequent and bad, tell your doctor. During late pregnancy this may be a sign of high blood pressure or some other complication.

Insomnia

Sometimes in late pregnancy, it can be difficult to get a good night's sleep. The discomfort is too much. Some women may have very vivid dreams during this period. Some of these dreams are rather unpleasant.

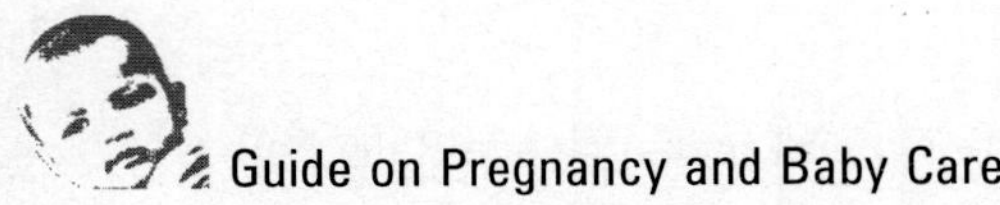

What to do

You should never let such dreams prey on your mind. Use lots of pillows. Try lying on one side with a pillow under your tummy and another under your top leg. If you cannot sleep well during the night, try to catch up on your rest during the day.

Fatigue

In the early months of pregnancy you may feel not just tired but desperately exhausted. It can be hard to handle–especially with young children or a tiring job.

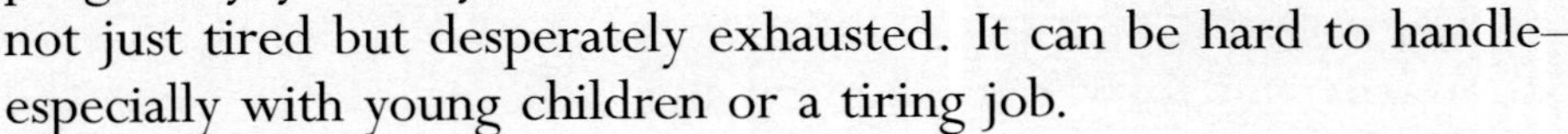

What to do

The only advice is to try to rest as much as you possibly can. Sometimes tiredness is the result of worry. If you know that you are worrying about something, it will help to talk about it–with your spouse, doctor, or a friend.

Breathlessness

It is common to feel breathless during pregnancy. That is because your body has to breath harder in order to eject the carbon dioxide that your baby produces and passes into your bloodstream via the placenta. In late pregnancy, the uterus also pushes the diaphragm up allowing less room for the lungs to expand.

What to do

If the breathlessness is accompanied by cough or chest pains, or episodes of fainting, then consult your doctor. If you have asthma, make sure that it is well controlled.Inhalers can be used safely all through pregnancy. In contrast, a bad asthma attack might reduce the baby's oxygen supply and can be dangerous.

Excessive urination

Needing to pass urine often is an early sign of pregnancy and for some women this condition can last until delivery. It is not known exactly what causes it in early pregnancy, but later it is the result of the womb pressing on the bladder.

What to do

In early pregnancy there is little you can do but put up with it. If it disturbs you to have to get up in the night, try drinking less liquid in the late evening. Later on some women find it helps to rock backwards and forwards while on the toilet seat. This eases the pressure of the womb on the bladder and you are more likely to empty it properly.

If you detect pain while passing urine, or pass blood, you may have a urinary infection. It is common to have cystitis in pregnancy. See your doctor about it.

Abdominal pain

Often abdominal pains up the sides of the womb are due to stretching of the ligaments. These are not serious. Some women experience a severe discomfort just in front of the bladder where the pubic bones meet in the mid-line. Usually these bones are held together tightly by a strong ligament, but in pregnancy this softens and stretches to make more space in the pelvis. This may be discomforting particularly while walking or exercising when the pubic bones tend to move in relation to each other.

What to do

There is no treatment and this will spontaneously settle after pregnancy. A caution: if the abdominal pain is severe or is accompanied by spotting or bleeding, you should immediately consult a doctor.

Constipation

Constipation is a common complaint during pregnancy due to the progesterone effect. Iron supplements may also add to the problem. But you must never take stimulant laxatives, including some over-the-counter preparations sold in the guise of ayurvedic pills, because they can sometimes stimulate the womb as well.

What to do

Include plenty of fibre in your diet. Your diet should include lots of fruits, vegetables, roti, wholemeal bread and high-fibre breakfast cereals. You should also have plenty of fluids. A simple laxative like lactulose may be useful occasionally. Some people find that a hot drink first thing in the morning also helps. If you continue to have constipation, you increase your risk of getting piles. As it is, the pressure of the growing baby on the blood vessels of the region increases the risk.

Piles

Piles is caused by constipation and straining. It also occurs in pregnancy because of hormonal changes. You can usually feel the

lumpiness of the piles around the back passage when you wash yourself after going to the loo, and they may ache a bit. The condition nearly always normalises within a week or two of delivery.

What to do

Eat plenty of food that is high in fibre to prevent constipation – roti, wholemeal bread, and fruit and vegetables. And avoid standing for long periods if you can. If the piles stick out, use a lubricating jelly and push them gently back inside. Your doctor can suggest an anaesthetic ointment for you.

Backache

From early months of pregnancy until about six months after the birth, you could suffer from backache. There are a number of possible causes. During pregnancy, the ligaments which support the spine become softened. There is also a shift in your centre of gravity as you get bigger. Sitting or standing badly can worsen the condition.

What to do

Most women can avoid bad back problems by following some simple guidelines: Adopt good posture habits:

- Do not lean backward while standing, even though you may feel comfortable that way. The correct standing posture is to stand straight, keeping the feet apart.
- Sit with your back supported
- While lifting or picking objects from the floor, avoid bending forward. Keeping the back straight, bend from the knees and then lift.
- Hold heavy objects close to your body
- Avoid stooping as for as possible

A firm mattress is very beneficial. If yours is soft, a piece of hardboard under the length of mattress will make it firmer.

Massage can also help to ease an aching back. Also in the later months ensure you get enough rest.

If the backache persists, talk to your doctor. A physiotherapist will also be able to give you advice and suggest some helpful exercises.

Cramps

Cramps are very common during pregnancy, and they can be very painful. They occur usually at night, in the legs or feet. The cause is not really known, but may be caused by lack of calcium. You, therefore, may need calcium supplements.

What to do

To treat cramps, rub the muscles very hard. It also helps to bend your foot upwards with your hand. Ask your spouse to do this for you if you cannot manage it. It may also help to go for a short walk or exercise your legs and feet in some other way just before going to bed to get the circulation going.

Bleeding Gums

Dental care should not be neglected during pregnancy. The cause of bleeding gums, whether you are pregnant or not, is the build-up of plaque (bacteria) on the teeth. This irritates the gums.

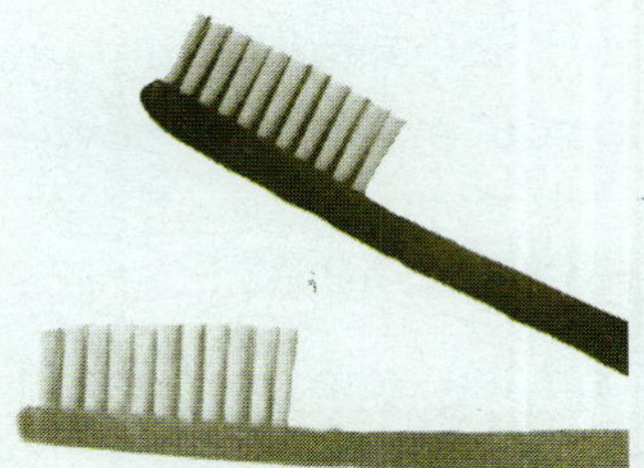

What to do

During pregnancy, pay special attention to cleaning your teeth. Brush really well, at least twice a day, before retiring at night and after breakfast, to remove all the plaque. Use a soft brush and teach yourself the correct method to brush.

Nose bleeds

Nosebleeds are quite common in pregnancy. Usually short, on occasions the bleeding can be quite heavy. So long as you do not lose a lot of blood, there is nothing to worry about. Blow your nose gently, and try to stifle sneezes.

What to do

To stop a bleed, pinch the nose. The bleeding will soon stop.

Itching

As your baby grows, the skin of your abdomen gets tighter and may itch a lot. There is little you can do about this, though it is very annoying.

What to do

It can help to wear smooth materials next to the skin, and to wear loose dresses so that there is no waistband to rub against you. Bathing also helps and some women find it soothing to apply hand cream or lotion or talcum powder.

Varicose veins

The leg veins can swell during pregnancy. This happens due to the pressure effect of the growing uterus on the pelvic veins. The good thing about them is that these often settle by themselves after childbirth and although uncomfortable, they do not usually bleed or thrombose.

What to do

The best way to control these is to avoid standing for long periods and not to sit with your legs crossed. Also do not put on more weight than you should. It can ease discomfort to sit with your legs up as often as you can, and to wear support tights. You can also try sleeping with your legs up on pillows, or even to raise the bottom end of your bed to keep your legs higher than the rest of your body.

Swelling in the ankles and feet

It is very common during the later part of pregnancy to have swelling in the ankles, feet and hands. This happens simply because the body holds more water than usual. Towards the end of the day, especially if the weather is hot or you have been standing a lot, the extra water tends to gather in the lowest parts of the body.

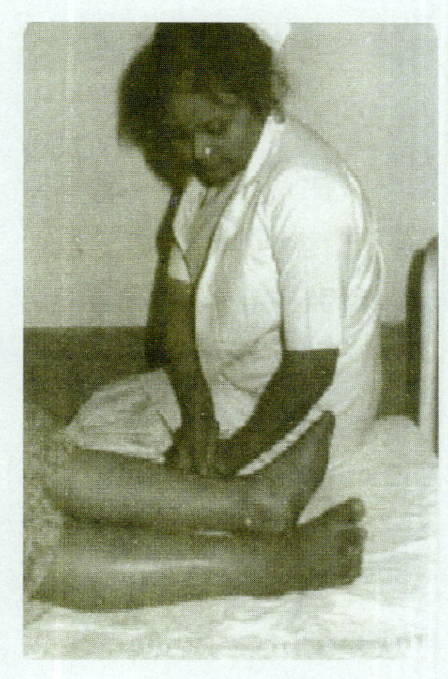

What to do

Wear comfortable sandals and shoes, and put your feet up as much as you can. Try to rest by lying flat in bed for at least one hour during the day. The important thing is to lie with your feet higher than your heart.

If your hands are getting puffy, take the rings off before they become stuck.

Occasionally some pregnant women develop a clot in the deep veins of the leg. This also may show up as swelling in the affected leg. So, if the swelling is limited to one leg and the calf muscles are hot and tender, consult your doctor.

You should also guard against a condition called pre-eclampsia. The other signs found in this condition are high blood pressure and protein in the urine. If you develop swelling in your ankles, feet or fingers, the safest course, therefore, is to check with your doctor.

Swelling and varicose veins of the vulva

The vulva is the area around the vaginal opening, including the clitoris and labia. It is normal for the vulva to look purple during pregnancy. Sometimes the vulva becomes swollen and you may get a very heavy feeling. This is because the pressure of the baby's head interferes with the flow of blood and the veins in the vulva become congested.

What to do

Take plenty of rest. The swelling usually goes within 24 hours of delivery.

Vaginal discharge

Almost all women have more vaginal discharge in pregnancy. So long as you are not sore or itching, it is quite normal.

What to do

It can help to wear cotton pants. And use a tampon if you need to. Soreness or irritation, or a coloured or smelly discharge, probably means you have some sort of vaginal infection. The commonest is candidiasis. It is a fungal infection which covers the vaginal wall with

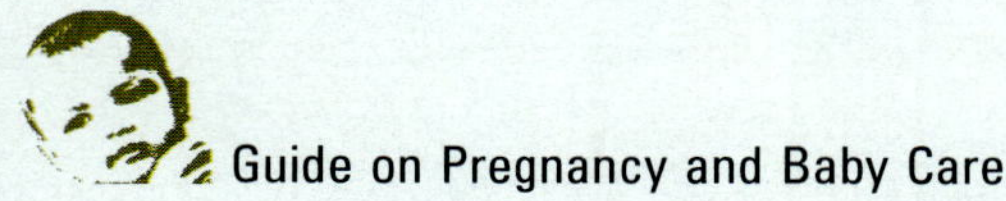

a white, curd-like material. The treatment is simple. There is rapid relief with anti fungal pessaries such as nystatin or clotrimazole vaginal tablets, one inserted each night as high in the vagina as possible. While nystatin must be used for 15 nights, a normal course of clotrimazole gets completed over six nights.

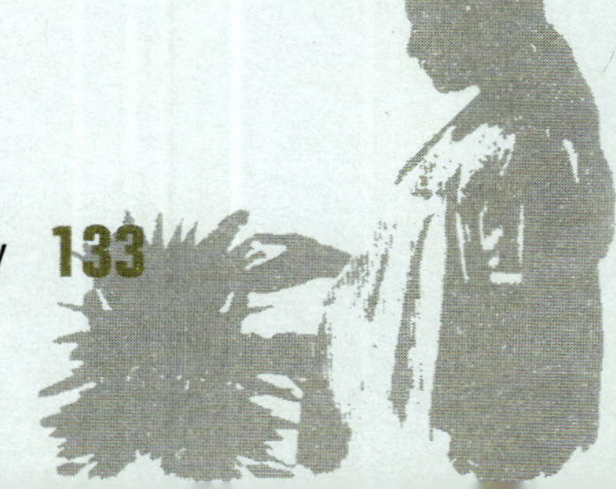

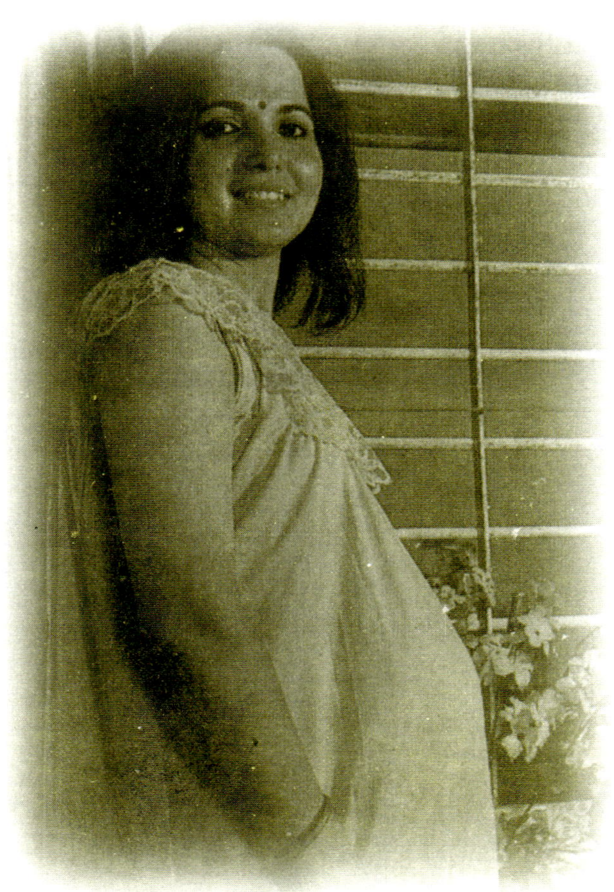

"It is odd but agitation or contest of any kind gives a rebound to my spirits and sets me up for a time."

-Lord Byron (1788-1824), English poet.
Letter, 8 March 1816, to poet Thomas Moore

Tiding Over The Difficult Problems

A number of difficult conditions can complicate pregnancy. Of them, anaemia is the commonest and easiest to treat. Urinary tract infection, toxaemia and premature rupture of membranes are all more difficult to handle. The emphasis should always be, therefore, on prevention. Good antenatal care consists of timely diagnosis and prompt treatment.

Anaemia

Anaemia, or deficiency of haemoglobin in the blood, is a common problem in pregnancy. Some anaemia is natural at this time, because the blood gets diluted due to increase in the liquid component of blood. But often the drop is more severe. If the haemoglobin level falls below 10 g per dl, it is a cause for concern. It calls for active treatment.

This deficiency of haemoglobin is rather common in Indian mothers, and the most common cause is iron deficiency. As pregnancy advances, more and more demands are made upon the mother's reserves of iron. During the last 12 weeks, baby's requirement of iron becomes very large. Unless the mother has been taking a healthy balanced diet with iron supplements and has sufficient stores of iron, the demand far exceeds the supply. In that case, mother's blood cells do not get sufficient iron and she develops anaemia. In many women, the shortfall occurs even before the pregnancy. A poor diet ensures the deficit, which is made worse by the menstrual loss.

Keeping a tab on haemoglobin level is an essential component of good antenatal care. You should undergo the haemoglobin test many times during pregnancy: at the first antenatal visit, then during the 28th week, and finally in the 36th week of gestation. This will allow you to take corrective steps on time. Unless the fall in haemoglobin is severe, you may not notice the symptoms. But if you feel any abnormal fatigue, a shortness of breath, paleness or swelling in the legs, think that it could be anaemia.

What to do

The best course, of course, is to take preventive steps. Never neglect to take the iron pills and capsules that the doctor writes for you. There are a number of preparations, and if one produces side effects, another can be tried. But if you have been careless and anaemia has set in, still there is no need to panic. Mild or moderate anaemia is mostly quick to respond to treatment. If however the deficiency is severe, then the deficit may have to be bridged by giving shots of iron. If the diagnosis is made in late pregnancy, it may need more concentrated effort. You may be given a total dose infusion of iron dextran through the veins.

In some mothers, the anaemia is compounded by a deficiency of folic acid. It is best therefore not to forget the folic acid pills. Be particular about them both during pregnancy and in the immediate period following your baby's birth.

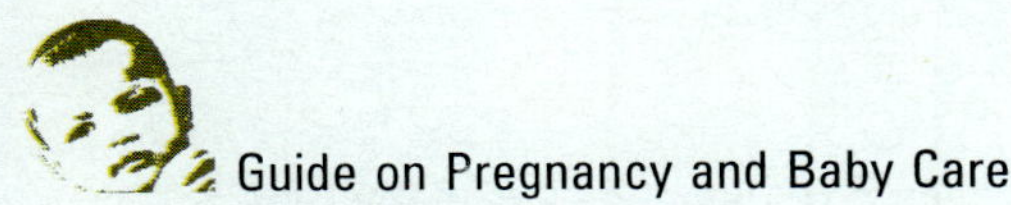

Urinary infections

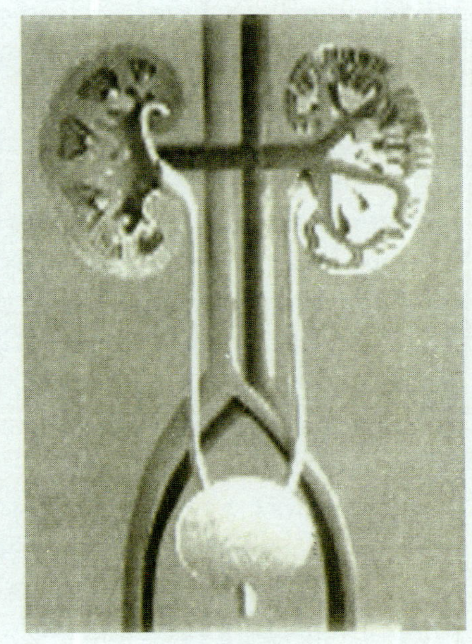

Infections of the bladder, and into the ureter and kidneys, are common during pregnancy. They can occur at any time, but are more common after the 20th week. These infections occur more easily during this period because of two factors. One, the enlarged uterus puts pressure on the ureter and this slows the flow of urine. Two, the pregnancy hormone (progesterone) causes a dilatation in the ureter which perhaps allows the infection to travel more easily to the kidneys. That's why once bacteria enter the bladder the infection is quick to spread into a full-blown urinary tract infection.

What to do

You must be quick to recognise the first symptoms. If you feel a burning or stinging while passing urine, visit the loo frequently, have fever with chills and suffer discomfort in the lower abdomen, it could be a urinary tract infection. See the doctor. You would need a urine test before starting the antibiotic treatment. You must also take complete bed rest and lots of liquids. Mostly, the treatment begins to show results within 48-72 hours. The fever comes down and the burning also stops. You must, however, continue the treatment for the prescribed period. Stopping the medicine without completing its course can lead to recurrence and a more difficult situation. The treatment usually lasts two weeks.

Toxaemia and eclampsia

Toxaemia or pre-eclampsia is a potentially serious complication of late pregnancy. The condition is marked by a sudden rise in blood pressure, rapid gain in weight from retention of fluid, swelling over the body and loss of protein in the urine. Its onset may be so quiet that it can catch you unawares. There may be a severe headache, pain in chest or upper abdomen, vomiting, drowsiness, dimness of vision and sudden swelling over the ankles, legs, abdomen, face, fingers and vulva.

In its more acute form, the onset is more dramatic and it rapidly passes into eclampsia. The mother has convulsions and she may go into coma. Her life is at serious risk and the baby may also die. In some instances, a premature labour may also set in.

Risk factors

Toxaemia is most common in first pregnancies. First-time mothers who are either less than 20 years old or over 35 years are the most likely sufferers. A mother who has suffered similarly during a previous pregnancy or has a mother or sister who suffered toxaemia is also at higher risk. The risk is also higher if there is a previous history of high blood pressure or kidney disease. A twin pregnancy and a small-statured mother also carry a higher than average risk.

Prevention

The best prevention against toxaemia is to be regular about the antenatal check ups. This way the condition can be diagnosed early. You must have a complete examination with weight and blood pressure and urine check up done on each visit.

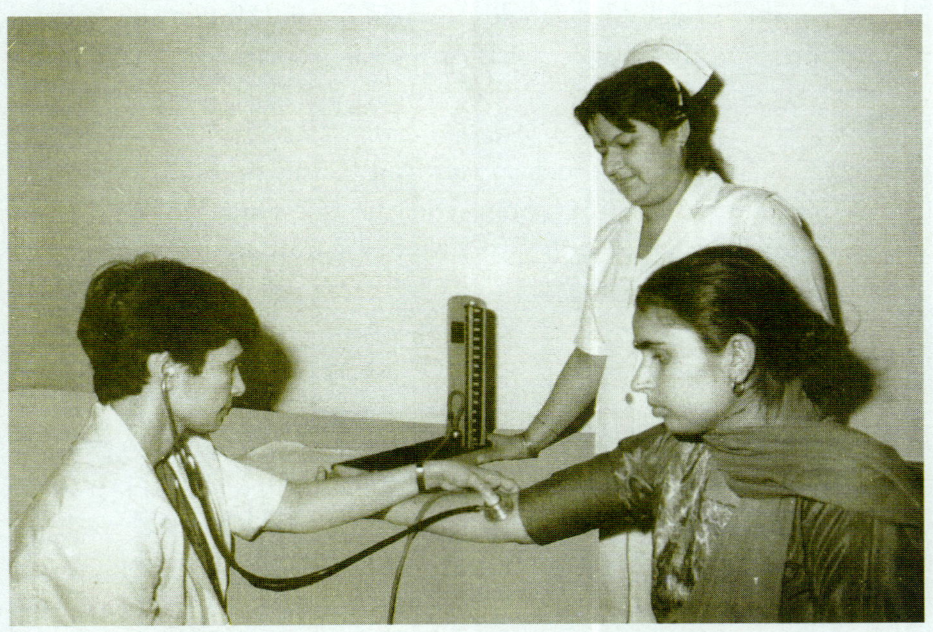

What to do

There is immediate need for specialist medical care. The mother must be admitted to a hospital immediately and put under close monitoring. She will need various forms of medication to control her symptoms. If this does not work, decision is taken to deliver the infant. This can save the situation many times and protect the life of both mother and child. The labour is either induced with the help of a intravenous drip or an emergency Caesarean section is done. If active treatment is not given, the condition carries a very high risk for the mother and baby.

Premature rupture of membranes

Sometimes the membranes around the baby rupture prematurely. This leads to a leakage of amniotic fluid through the vagina. In most instances, this is followed quickly by childbirth. Unless the baby is mature enough, the chances of his survival are slim.

Causes

A number of mechanical factors can lead to this premature rupture of membranes. For instance, the cervix can be loose and incompetent or too much fluid may accumulate in the bag of membranes or a twin pregnancy can lead to an increased tension on the uterus.

Prevention

If the cervix is incompetent, the problem is likely to recur. To prevent this, some obstetricians apply a special stitch during early pregnancy on the cervix. The procedure is known as the McDonald's stitch. This stitch is subsequently removed at the time of delivery.

What to do

The obstetrician must be informed immediately. Generally once the membranes rupture, it is difficult to stop labour. In more than 80 per cent cases, the mother goes into labour within the next 24 hours. That means all efforts must centre on taking the baby to a nursery which has arrangements to care for a premature infant.

But if labour does not supervene and the pregnancy is much under 36 weeks, an all-out effort is made to delay the onset of labour. The mother is put under complete bed rest and medications are given in an attempt to suppress labour. She must also wear a sterile pad over the vulva so that bacteria may not find entrance into the uterus. The baby also has to be kept under a constant watch. He is at risk because the cord can get compressed and this can lead to a compromised blood supply and also, sometimes due to infection.

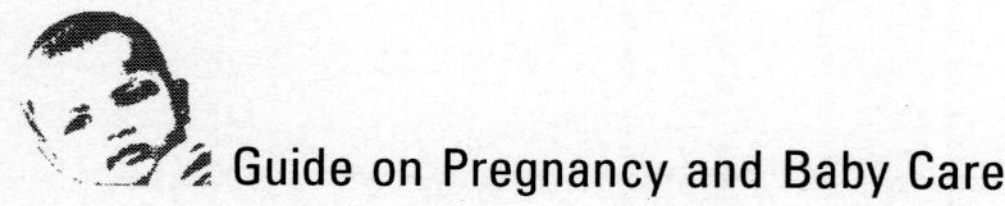

That's why, if the pregnancy has advanced to 36 weeks or more, and labour does not set in spontaneously, attempt is made to deliver the baby as soon as possible. If the baby's heart rate shows a sudden slowing or irregularity, and the pelvic examination shows a decrease in amniotic fluid, immediate delivery alone can save the baby. This may mean a Caesarean section.

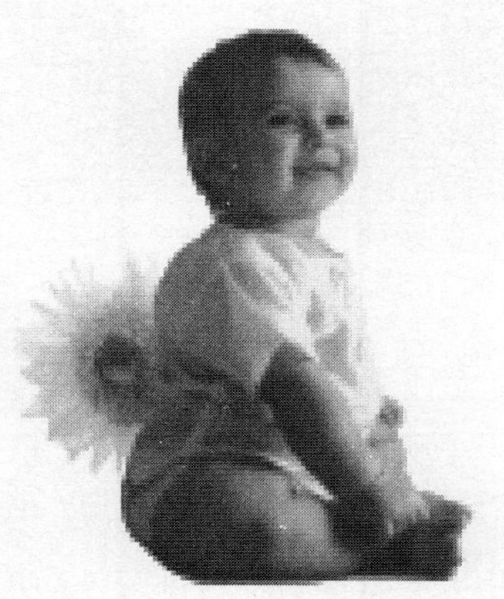

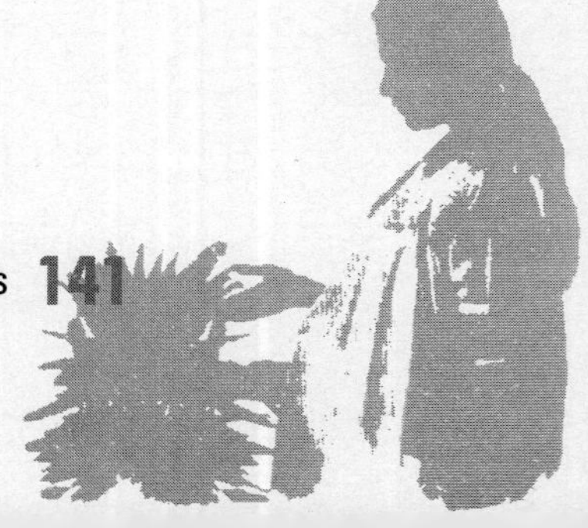

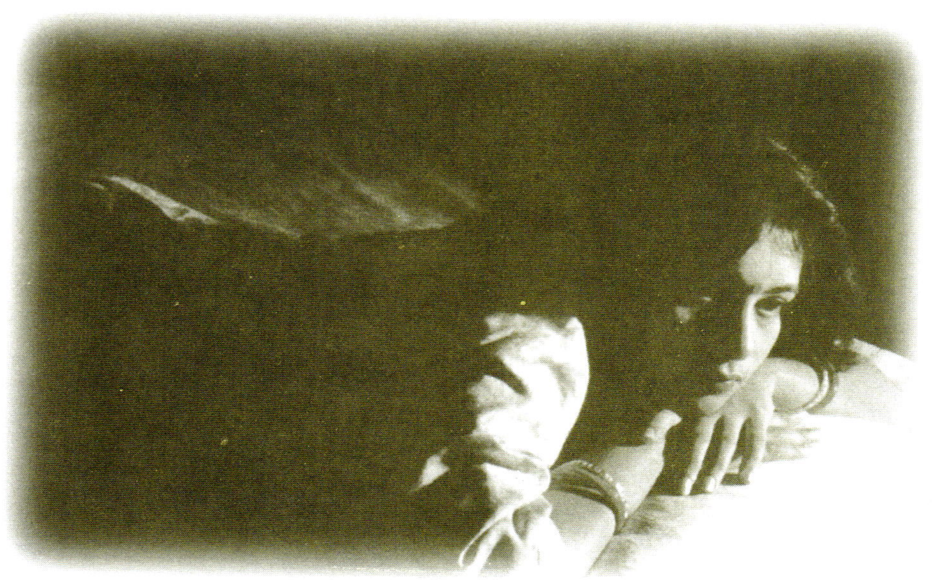

*"Ah, Hope! what would life be,
stripped of thy encouraging smiles,
that teach us to look behind the dark clouds of today,
for the golden beams that are to gild the morrow."*

-Susanna Moodie (1803-85), Canadian author.
Life in the Clearing

When Pregnancy Goes Wrong

Most pregnancies happily go to term without mishap. But occasionally pregnant women have to bear with some complications that need intensive care or supervision of obstetrician. Nearly 15 per cent of pregnancies go waste. Disappointment is very natural at this stage, but the mission is to save the mother's life. Even though the movie world makes us believe that there are situations when either the baby or mother can survive, in real life it is only the mother who can benefit with prompt medical care and attention. We also discuss the poignant situation when the newborn baby is handicapped.

Miscarriage

A miscarriage can be very difficult to come to terms with. You may feel angry, or guilty, wondering what you did wrong. You will almost certainly feel a sense of loss. You will need to grieve over the lost baby just as you would over the death of anyone close to you, especially if the miscarriage has happened in advanced pregnancy. Remember, it is not the end of the road for you.

Causes

Miscarriages are, in fact, quite common, especially before 12 weeks. There are reasons to believe that at least one in six pregnancies end in this way. At this early stage a miscarriage usually happens because there is something wrong with the fertilised egg. Often, it has a genetic fault and it is best it ends this way. Sometimes, the embedding of the egg does not happen properly, and it aborts. A later miscarriage can be due to the placenta not working properly, or the cervix being weak and opening too early. A serious illness such as severe high blood pressure, toxaemia, sexually transmitted diseases such as caused by cytomegalovirus, the herpes simplex virus, and Mycoplasma hominis, and defects in the endocrine glands can also cause a miscarriage.

Whatever the cause, a miscarriage is rarely anyone's fault. Many people believe that making love during pregnancy can cause a miscarriage. This is very unlikely. If a couple make love and then soon after the woman has a miscarriage, it may seem as though intercourse was the cause. As a result many couples blame themselves when there is no reason for them to do so.

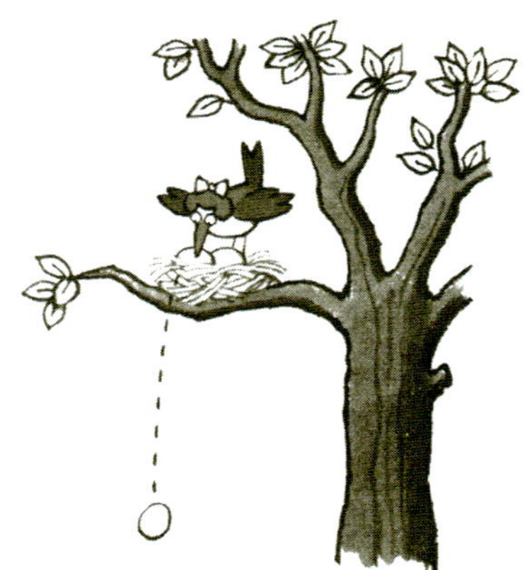

Many couples ask the question of how certain activities or a person's life-style may affect the risk of miscarriage. With increasing numbers of women taking up jobs, the affect of work on pregnancy is one such area of concern. In general, women who wish to work may continue do so, close to or actually up to the end of their pregnancy, if they feel well and have no medical contraindications.

Physical exercise is another concern. While a certain amount of exercise is good for all healthy pregnant women, there is, obviously, a need not to overdo it. Pointing fingers have also been raised on trivial physical trauma such as travelling in a rickety bus. Sometimes, a woman remembers a minor accident that immediately precedes miscarriage and concludes a cause-and-effect relationship. However, there are many documented cases in which severe trauma, such as multiple fractures of the pelvis, has occurred without an interruption of the pregnancy.

Symptoms and Signs

A miscarriage is a 'natural abortion'. It is the ending of a pregnancy before the 28th week. After the 28th week, a baby has a good chance of survival if it is delivered.

An early miscarriage often happens around the time that you would have expected to have a period. It can be rather like a period, with bleeding and a similar sort of aching pain. A later miscarriage after the first three months, is more like labour itself. That's because by now the foetus has taken form.

Any bleeding in pregnancy could be the start of a miscarriage. If you begin to bleed, consult your doctor as soon as you can—immediately if you are losing a lot of blood. You will probably be advised to go to bed and rest. In about 50 per cent women who experience bleeding and cramps early in pregnancy the bleeding will stop and the pregnancy will carry on quite normally. But in other cases the miscarriage in inevitable.

That is called an inevitable abortion. In such case, the bleeding becomes heavier and cramps are more severe. On examination, the doctor may be able to feel the cervix beginning to open up and dilate and the products of conception lying at the external opening of the cervix. At this time the changes that have occurred are irreversible, and no therapy will prevent the abortion.

Sometimes the miscarriage is incomplete, and the entire products of conception are not expelled. Such an incomplete abortion particularly happens in pregnancies beyond the sixth and up to the 14th week. Very often the foetal tissues are unrecognisable

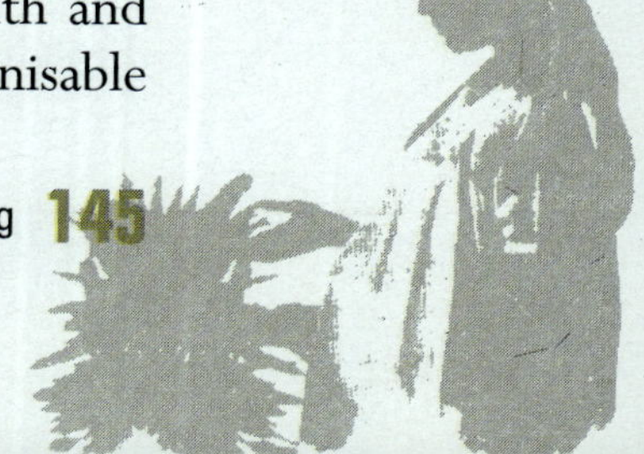

because foetal death occurred a number of days or weeks before expulsion. In this case cramping will range from moderate to severe, and bleeding may be very extensive and actually life-threatening. Bleeding will continue until all of the remaining placental tissue is removed. The uterus will be able to contract only then, cutting off the blood vessels that are producing the haemorrhage.

Occasionally, the fertilised egg stops growing and dies but, for some unknown reason, labour does not ensue immediately. This is a missed abortion. In this type of abortion, the foetus may remain in the uterine cavity, sometimes for as long as eight weeks. There is usually a clinical history of early bleeding that stops spontaneously or after some form of therapy. However, the breasts revert back to the non-pregnant state, and the size of the uterus not only ceases to increase, but actually decreases with time.

Treatment

After a miscarriage, your doctor would take you in for a cleaning job. This simple operation is called a 'D & C' that is, dilation and curettage. Its aim is to clean the womb. The cervix is gently opened and the lining of the womb scraped or sucked away. At the same time, medication in given to help the uterus contract so that the bleeding stops.

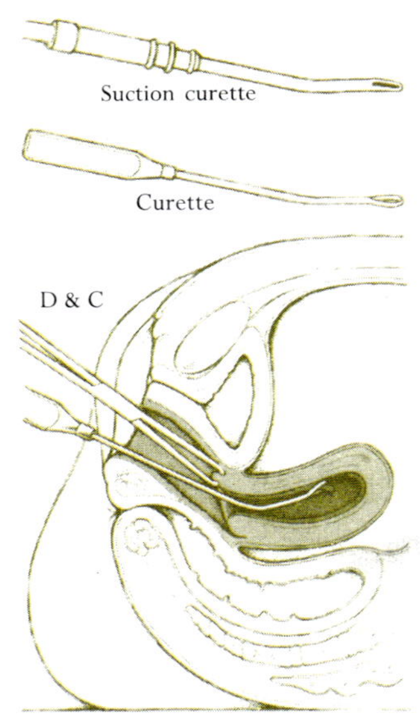

At this point it is very important to remember that if the mother is Rhesus negative, she is given the anti-D shot. Failure to do so may result in Rhesus sensitivity, which could affect future pregnancies and cause blood incompatibility (mismatch) between the mother and foetus leading to serious complications.

The future

A miscarriage does not mean that you will be unable to have children. In fact, if you have only had one miscarriage, you have a very good chance of having a success-ful pregnancy next time. It is up to you whether you try to get pregnant again now or after a while.

Ectopic Pregnancy

Sometimes a pregnancy goes wrong at the very onset. After conception, the fertilised egg, instead of moving into the womb, gets stuck in the fallopian tube and begins to grow there. Much less commonly, the fertilisation occurs in the ovary or the egg reaches the cervical canal. On rare occasions the egg is either fertilised outside the tube or discharged from the free end of the tube after fertilisation; it then gets implanted within the abdominal cavity, establishes a blood supply, and continues to develop. Such pregnancies usually do not survive, although in extremely rare cases

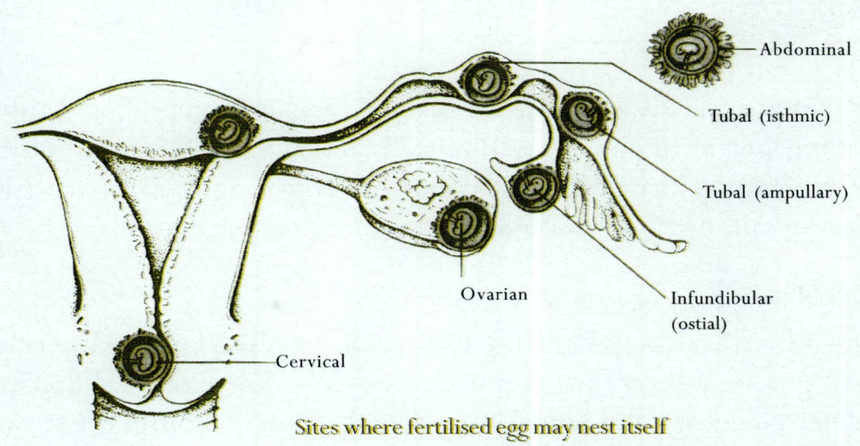

Sites where fertilised egg may nest itself

they actually go to term. All of them make for an ectopic (out of place) pregnancy.

Causes

A common cause of an ectopic pregnancy is a blockage or an infection in the fallopian tube. For example, the tube may have been damaged by an infection. This produces structural distortion of the tubes. The sperms can move up to the free end of the tube, near the ovary where fertilization occurs, but the passage is too narrow to permit the fertilised egg to make its way into the womb cavity. There may be number of other factors also. These include a history of a previous

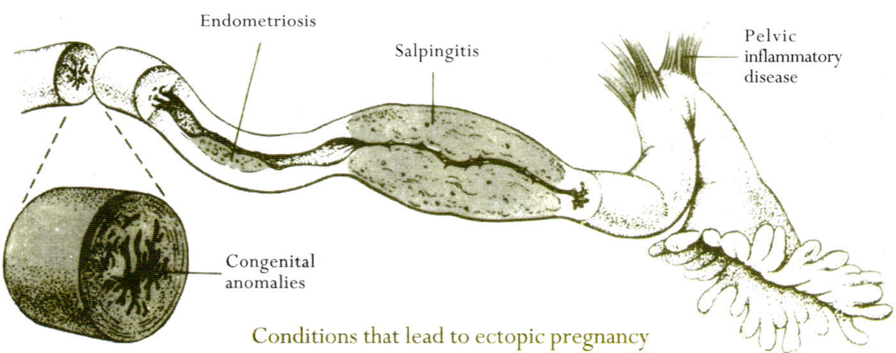

Conditions that lead to ectopic pregnancy

ectopic pregnancy, a Caesarean section, pelvic surgery, failed tubal ligation, pelvic tumours, and induced and spontaneous abortion or use of fertility drugs or post-coital oestrogen contraceptives (the morning-after pill) or an existing endometriosis.

Symptoms

Signs of an ectopic pregnancy usually occur after a missed period. The signs are a severe pain on one side—low down in the abdomen, vaginal bleeding, and sometimes feeling faint. If you get a strong one-sided pain and it is possible that you may be pregnant, do not delay. Contact the doctor immediately. There is a serious risk that the bleeding may become so severe that it may lead to shock.

Diagnosis

When all of the signs and symptoms of ruptured ectopic pregnancy are present, the doctor can diagnose the condition rather comfortably. However, an early diagnosis, prior to rupture, is difficult. Before the pregnancy achieves a certain size, it may be difficult or even impossible for the physician to feel. Further, similar symptoms can occur in a number of conditions. These include pelvic inflammatory disease, endometriosis, rupture or twisting of an ovarian cyst, and spontaneous miscarriage.

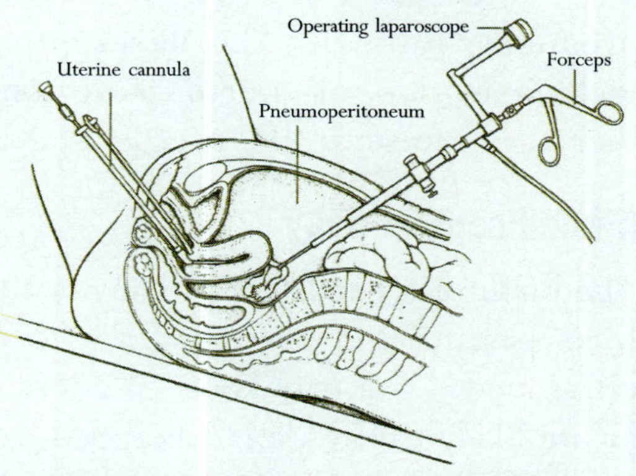

Laparascopy is the best way to diagnose an ectopic pregnancy

The way to an early diagnosis is through the ultrasound and hormonal pregnancy tests. These tests, however, are not totally infallible. That is why doctors sometimes do culdocentesis. In this pro-cedure a hollow needle is inserted into the lower pelvic cavity through the upper vagina. If there is internal bleeding, blood will be aspirated from this space; and this would support the possibility of an ectopic pregnancy. In some cases however, it becomes necessary to perform an immediate laparoscopic examination. Using a slender, tubular endoscope inserted through an incision in the abdominal wall, the surgeon examines the pelvic cavity in detail.

Treatment

The treatment for ectopic pregnancy depends on the site it has implanted and on the patient's condition. Needless to say, it calls for an immediate hospitalisation, blood transfusions and surgery. Most surgeons prefer a conservative approach and try to preserve a woman's child bearing ability whenever possible, particularly if the patient is childless, has fertility problems, or is quite young. It is increasingly common, when the pregnancy has not yet ruptured, for the doctor to open the tube surgically, remove the pregnancy, and close the tube, leaving it in place. In the past when a woman had to have both tubes removed, the uterus was usually removed as well, since there was no longer a possibility of her becoming pregnant. But with the development of in vitro fertilisation techniques this, of course, is no longer the case, and physicians therefore, preserve the uterus.

A handicapped baby

The birth of a handicapped baby is an extremely difficult situation. Most parents find it very hard to cope, even though—because of ultrasound—you may know in advance that you are going to have, or are likely to have, a handicapped baby. Sometimes you may come to know only some months after, when the baby does not show optimum progress in his development.

Many parents, and mothers in particular, have to cope with feelings of guilt and the idea that in some way they have caused their baby's problem. This feeling of guilt is almost always unjustified, but that does not make it less real. It will take time, and the right people around you, and probably a lot of talking, before you can feel better. It is certainly not the time to point accusing fingers at each other.

What to do

It is a responsibility you have been given, and it is your duty to do your best. The need is to get as much support and information as you possibly can. Your treating obstetrician and baby's paediatrician, and your family physician may be able to help in this regard. You would have to look for and find what best help is available in your neighbourhood for your baby, and what treatment opportunities exist. Many children with a handicap do better than able-bodied people given proper support and surroundings. The idea should be to find the best possible treatment for them and not think of them as a burden or punishment. A positive and caring attitude can see them grow well and happily.

It may also be a good idea to see a genetic counsellor who has special knowledge about the reasons why such handicap occur and what would be the chances, if any, that the defect may recur in a subsequent child.

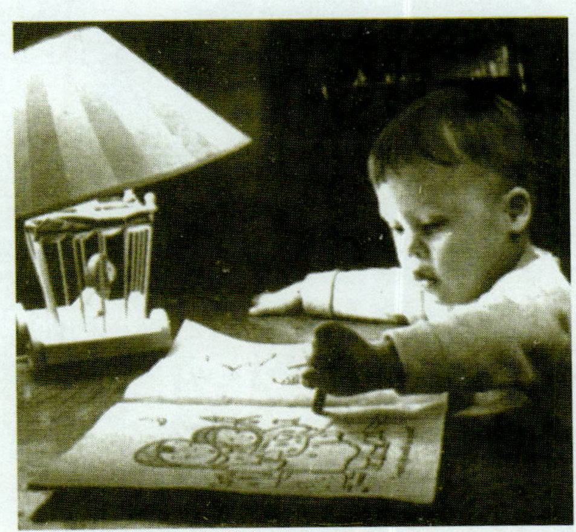

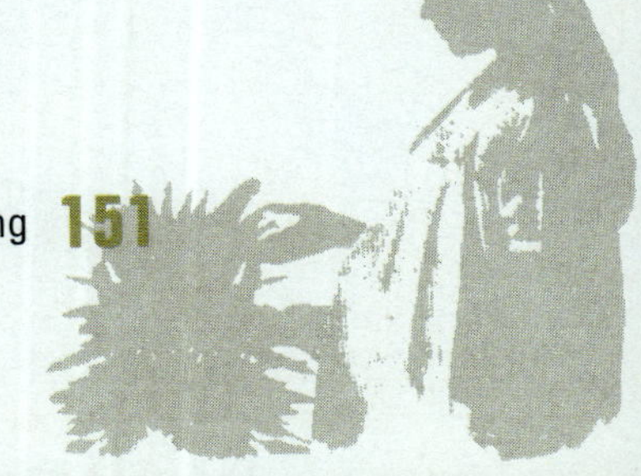

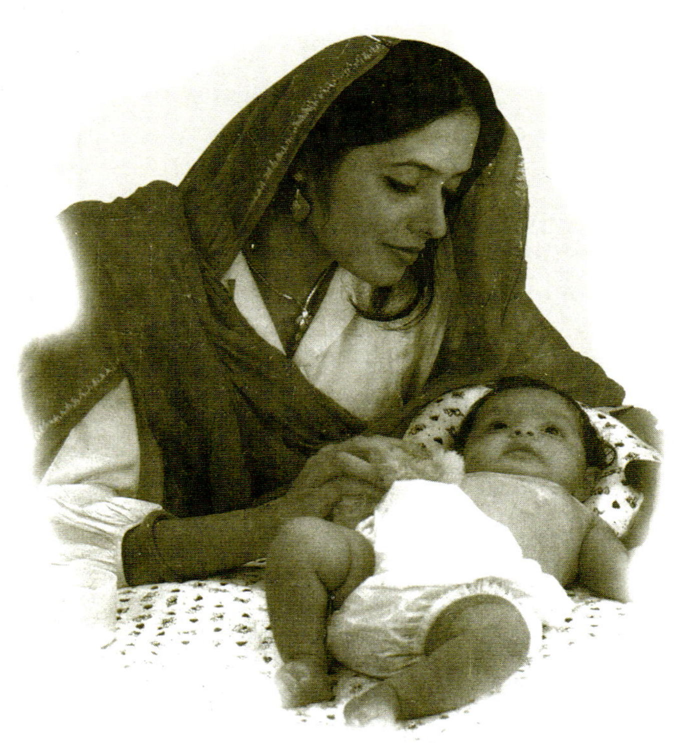

"A woman when she is in travail hath sorrow,
because her hour is come:
but as soon as she is delivered of the child,
she remembereth
no more the anguish,
for joy that a man is born into the world."

-Bible: New Testament. John 16:21.

Welcoming Your Baby

Delivery, the process by which the baby is expelled from the uterus through the birth canal and into the world, begins with irregular contractions of the uterus that occur every 20 to 30 minutes. As labour progresses, the contractions increase in frequency and severity. The usual length of labour for a first-time mother is about 13 to 14 hours, and about 8 or 9 hours in a woman who has given birth previously. Wide variations exist, however, in the duration of labour.

Preparing for birth

There are some things you need to do before your baby is due.

Pack a case a few weeks ahead ready to take into hospital with you. You will need:

1. Night clothes—front opening if you are going to breastfeed
2. Dressing gown and slippers
3. Nursing bras—or ordinary bras
4. Pyjamas, and a belt, to hold sanitary towels in place
5. Toilet bag—hairbrush, towel, toothbrush, etc
6. Nappies and other things needed for the baby

If you already have children, make suitable arrangements for who will look after them when you go into hospital. It may even be the middle of the night. If possible, it should also be someone your child knows. Once you have made this arrangement, and if your child is old enough, talk to him or her about what will happen.

Keep a list of the important telephone numbers at hand such as that of your doctor, the hospital or the nursing home, your husband's, a friend or close relative who can be called in an emergency. Keep the numbers handy so that when you go into labour, you do not have to look them up.

Work out how you will get to the hospital when the time comes. If you do not have a car, you should think what would be the best alternative. If you are going by car, make sure there is always enough petrol in the tank.

Think ahead to the time when you come out of hospital and make whatever plans you can. For example, neither you nor whoever is looking after you will want to do much shopping. So stock up on things like dry rations, washing powder and other groceries. Make sure you have got in the essentials for the baby: nappies, clothes etc. Buy some sanitary towels as you will have a discharge for up to two weeks after the birth and it will probably be quite heavy at first.

Pack a bag ready for coming out of hospital with some loose, easy-to-wear clothes for you, baby clothes, a couple of spare nappies, and if it is cold, a shawl or blanket to wrap the baby in.

How to recognise when the labour starts

Throughout pregnancy, the muscles of the womb contract, practising for labour. In the last weeks of pregnancy you will probably notice these contractions happening more often. Your abdomen will get hard and then relax again. These contractions, called Braxton Hicks' contractions, are usually painless and quite different from the contractions that happen in labour.

Many women worry that they may not recognise the beginning of labour, but you are unlikely to mistake the signs when the time really comes. You are more likely to make a mistake if labour starts early, before you expect it.

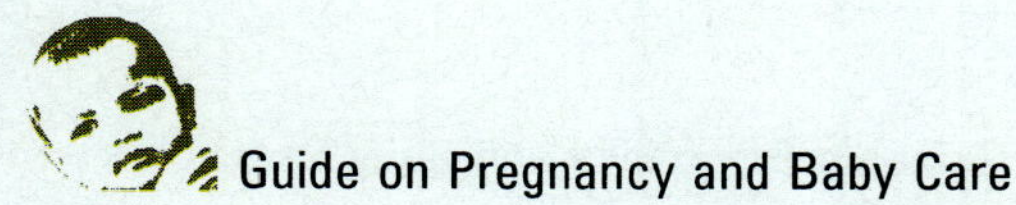

Remember that some women do go into labour early–maybe even some weeks before they are due. If you get pains in your abdomen that you have not had before, or a backache, which seems different from any backache you have had in pregnancy, or if you start losing blood or your waters break, then contact your doctor.

The signs that labour is beginning are:

Regular contractions

At first you may get very mild contractions. Your back may ache, or you may get the aching, heavy feeling that for some women goes with a monthly period. You may feel queasy or have diarrhoea. Time the spaces between contractions. Gradually the contractions will grow stronger and occur more often. When they are coming regularly, about every 10 or 15 minutes, or when you feel you can no longer cope on your own, it is time to call the hospital and to go in. If you live a long way from the hospital, or if this is not your first baby, it is better to go earlier rather than later.

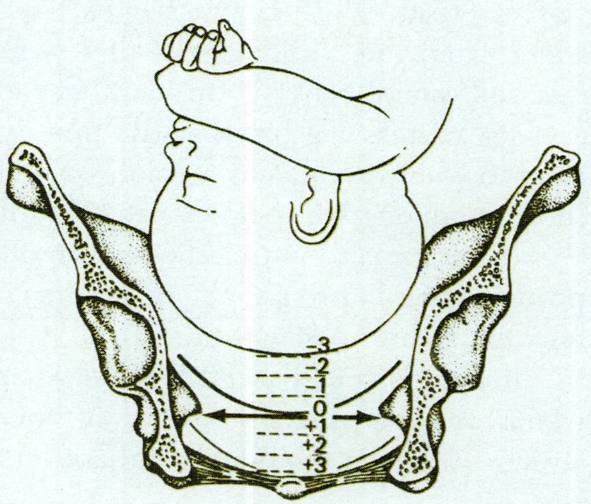

'Show'

Either before labour starts, or sometimes during the first stage of labour, the plug of mucus in the neck of the womb breaks away and is passed out of the vagina. This is called a 'show'. If it happens before

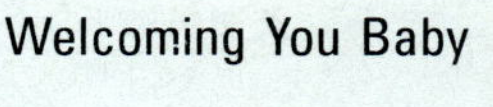

you go into labour, you may notice it as just a small amount of sticky, pinkish mucus.

You normally do not lose a lot of blood with a 'show'–just a little, mixed with the mucus. If you are losing more blood, it is a sign that something is wrong. It is time to move to the hospital or nursing home to be with your obstetrician.

The waters breaking

The bag of water in which the baby is floating may break at the beginning of labour or not until labour is well under way. If the waters break before labour begins, you will notice either a slow trickle from your vagina or else there will be a sudden gush of water that you cannot control. Go in at once to the hospital.

The waters can break at any time without warning. If you are close to your date of delivery and you are going out, a sanitary towel (not a tampon) will help to catch the flow if your waters should break. You can also put plastic underneath the sheet on your bed to protect your mattress, but in summer this can be quite hot and uncomfortable to sleep on.

If you are at all uncertain about whether or not you are starting labour, or about whether or not it is time for you to go into hospital, always telephone the doctor and ask for advice.

At the hospital

Hospitals vary, so this is just a guide to what is likely to happen. It is a good idea to find out in advance about the way things are done at your hospital. Just as important, think in advance about the way you yourself would like things to be done. You should always ask for what you want, and if your wishes cannot be met, it is important to understand why.

The obstetrician will examine you and ask you about what has been happening so far. She will take your pulse, temperature and blood pressure and check your urine. She will feel your abdomen to find out the baby's position, and listen to the baby's heart. She will probably also do an internal examination to find out how much your cervix has opened. Tell the obstetrician if a contraction is coming so she can wait until it has passed before she does the examination. She will then be able to tell you how far your labour has progressed. Ask about anything you want to know.

Your pubic hair may be shaved. Some hospitals do not shave at all. Many shave away just the hair round the vaginal opening.

The obstetrician may also put a suppository into your back passage or give you an enema. Within a few minutes you will be able to go to the lavatory and empty your bowels. A suppository or enema is not always needed. A lot of women find they empty their bowels naturally and easily before labour begins.

At some hospitals you may be given a bath. A warm bath can be soothing in the early stages of labour.

Next, you will go either straight to your own delivery room or to a first-stage labour ward, depending on how far the labour has progressed. If you go to a ward first, you will be moved to a delivery room when your baby is ready to be born.

Pain relief

As you get further into labour, the contractions become painful. During pregnancy you need to think and talk to your obstetrician about how you will cope. It is important to know what kinds of pain relief are available.

What you can do for yourself

There is no doubt that if you understand what's happening in labour, you will be better able to cope. Fear makes pain worse, and everybody feels frightened of what they do not understand or cannot control. So learning about labour and how to relax and breathe properly at antenatal classes can help a lot. It is possible to learn ways of breathing that make it possible for you to 'ride over' contractions, and concentrate on your breathing to take your mind off the pain.

It is also very important for you to feel in control of what is happening to you. So throughout your labour, do not hesitate to ask questions and to ask for whatever you want. You are working with the doctor, and she with you.

As well as relaxation and breathing, your posture can also make a difference. Kneeling helps some women, for example. Walking around, or moving in other ways such as rocking backwards and forwards, can also help. So can massage.

A great many women manage better in labour if someone whom they feel they can lean on, is with them. Most Indian hospitals, public hospitals included, do not allow any family member into the labour room. This should change. In the developed world, it is rather common for the spouse to be with the mother at childbirth.

Injections

Another form of pain relief is the injection of a medicine. The medications most widely used are pethidine and phenergan. The injections are easily and quickly given. They take about 20 minutes to work, and then the effects last for about two to four hours. For most women, these medications or similar others do lessen pain but do not do away with it altogether. The disadvantages of injected Medicines are that they can make you feel 'woozy'. You may feel drowsy so that you cannot push so well when you need to. Also, although there are no serious side effects, if you are given a medication like pethidine in the hour or so immediately before delivery, then your baby may be rather sleepy and a little slow to breathe at the time of birth. This however should not be a worrying thought because it can be taken care of very quickly.

Epidural block

An epidural is a special type of local anaesthetic. It numbs the nerves which carry the feelings of pain from the birth canal to the brain. So for most women an epidural gives complete pain relief.

An epidural has to be given by an anaesthetist. You lie curled up on one side and a needle is injected between the bones of your spine. A plastic tube is threaded down the needle into a place outside the nerves of the spinal cord. Then the needle is taken out. The tube is held in place on your back by a piece of sticking plaster. All this takes about 20 minutes. The anaesthetic is then injected down the tube and, as the effect of the first shot wears off, further 'top-up' injections can be given in the same way. The anaesthetic starts to work in about 15 to 20 minutes.

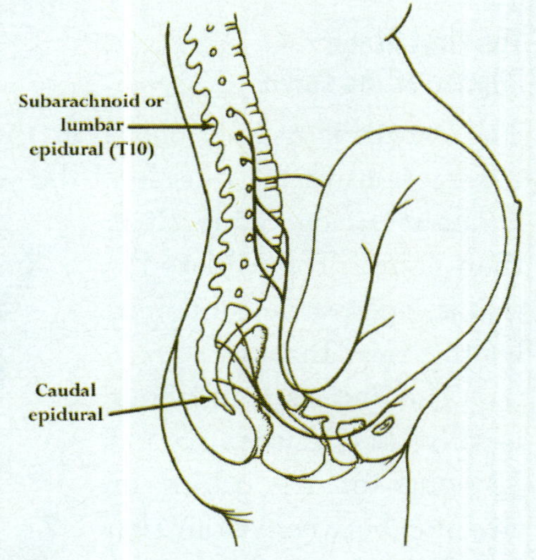

There are, however, some disadvantages too. Your legs feel heavy and lifeless, and that can make you feel rather dependent. You may find it difficult to pass urine on your own and it is difficult to move about. Also, since you can no longer feel your contractions, the obstetrician has to tell you when to push rather than you doing it naturally. This means that it can take longer to push the baby out. There is also a small but real risk of a sudden drop in blood pressure and infection. But in good hands, and with proper technique, the risk is very small.

What happens during labour

There are three stages to labour. In the first stage, the cervix gradually opens up (dilates). In the second stage, the baby is pushed down the vagina and is born. And in the third stage the placenta comes away from the wall of the womb and is pushed out of the vagina.

The First Stage
Dilation of The Cervix

The cervix is usually closed at the start of labour. Gradually the contractions of the muscle of the womb open up the cervix until it is about 10 cm wide. It is then called 'fully dilated'– that is, open wide enough to let the baby through.

The first stage of labour usually lasts between six and 12 hours for first babies, or anything between about two and seven hours for second and later babies. You can be up and moving about for most of the first stage if you feel like it.

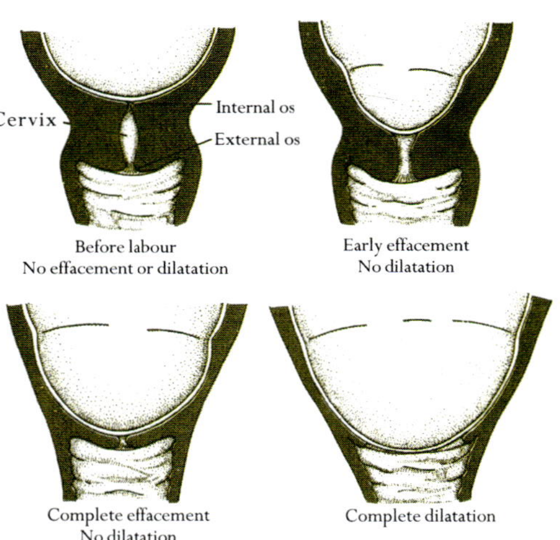

The uterine cervix widens and dilates to allow childbirth during the first stage

There may be times when you think nothing is happening. Ask the obstetrician to tell you how you are getting on.

You will probably be told not to eat anything so as to avoid being sick later in labour and also just in case an anaesthetic should be needed.

From time to time, the obstetrician will check how you are getting on. She will examine you to see how far the cervix has dilated and check the baby's heartbeat. The obstetrician may not stay with you all the time. You will be able to call her if you need her.

Gradually, the contractions will get stronger and more painful. The relaxation and breathing learnt during pregnancy can now be most helpful. Towards the end of the first stage, as each contraction comes, you may begin to feel that you want to push. At this point, the obstetrician should be back with you. She will tell you to try not to push until your cervix is fully open and the baby's head can be seen. To help yourself get over the urge to push, try blowing out gently and slowly, or if the urge is strong, in little puffs.

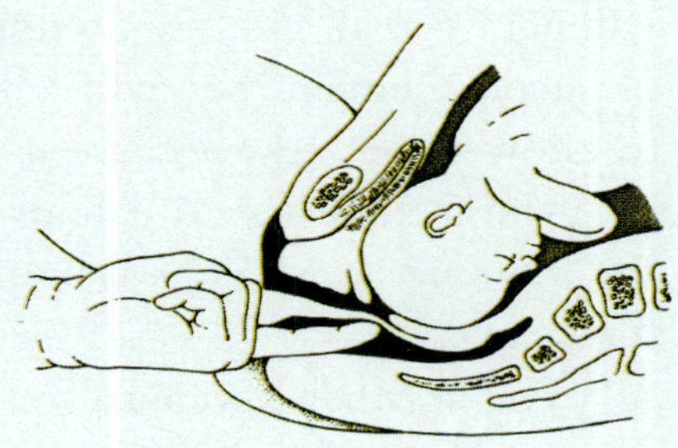

The Second Stage

Baby's Birth

The second stage is the descent of the baby and its actual birth. As soon as the cervix is wide enough, the contractions change their nature and become more purposeful, and you instinctively help by pushing. The muscle fibres of the uterus remain a little shorter after each contraction, and the baby is pushed down the vagina. There are just two obstacles: a sharp bend forwards from uterus to vagina, and the muscles, connective tissue and skin of the floor of the pelvis at the outlet from the vagina, which take some time to stretch. With some effort, you can overcome them.

The doctor will tell you when your cervix is fully dilated and your baby's head is showing. You can then start to push each time you have a contraction.

Find the position that suits you best. You may find that you want your back propped up, or to kneel on all fours, to lie on your side, or to squat. It is up to you. As the contraction starts, take two or three breaths and push down. Take another breath when you need to. Give several pushes until the contraction ends. As you push let yourself 'open up' below. After each contraction, rest and get up strength for the next one. This stage is hard work, but your doctor will help you all the time, telling you what to do and giving you lots of encouragement. She will tell you how you are doing. If you want to know more, ask, because it helps to know what's happening.

The second stage of labour can last for one or maybe two hours, but this varies a lot. The baby's head moves down the vagina until it 'crowns'.

This is when about half of the head can be seen at the vaginal opening. Then the doctor will tell you to push very gently, and to take quick short breaths through the mouth. This is so that your baby's head can emerge slowly. The skin, soft tissues and muscles of the perineum—the area between your vagina and back passage—are put to considerable stress as the baby's head emerges. If the head comes down too quickly, the tissue and the muscles sometimes undergo a tear. This tear may also sometimes run so far back as to

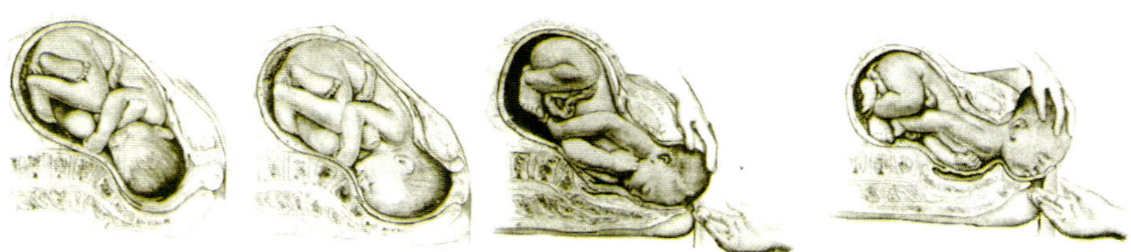

affect the anal sphincter. On the other hand, if the head descends in a more controlled manner, the vaginal opening has a better chance to stretch. A tear can thus be avoided.

Sometimes the skin of the perineum does not stretch enough. The doctor will then give you a local anaesthetic and cut the skin. This is called an episiotomy.

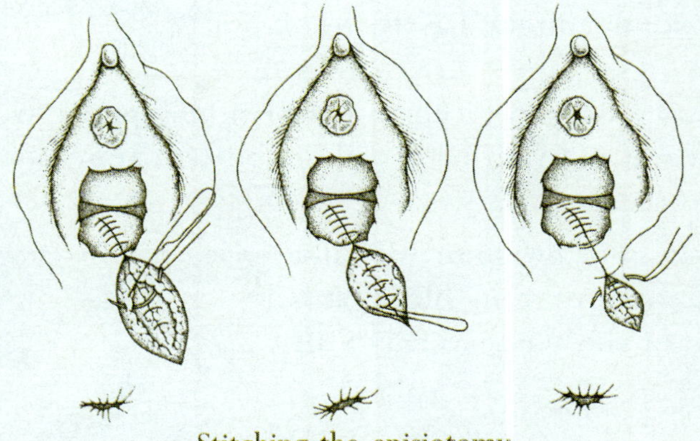

Stitching the episiotomy

Afterwards the cut is stitched up again and heals.

As your baby's head 'crowns', you can put your hand down and feel the head if you want to. Or if your doctor is a little innovative, she may show it with a mirror! Once the head is out, most of the hard work is over. With one more gentle push the rest of the body emerges quite quickly and easily.

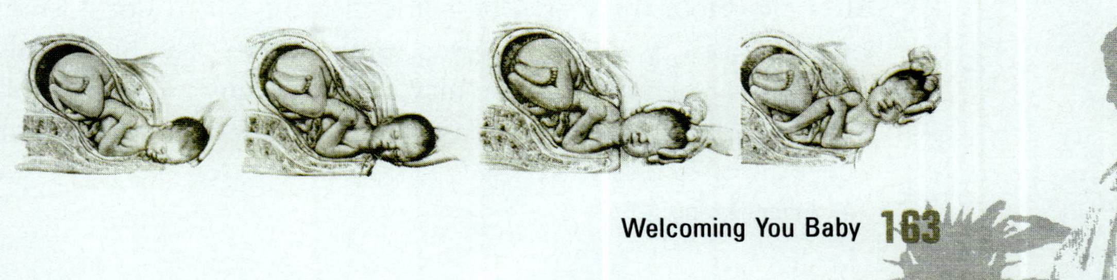

Usually your baby is lifted onto you, still attached by the cord, so that you can feel and be close to each other straight away. Then, as soon as the baby is breathing well, the cord is clamped and cut and you will be able to hold and cuddle your baby properly. Sometimes some mucus has to be cleared out of a baby's nose and mouth, or some oxygen given to get breathing under way. This is not at all unusual and your baby will not be kept away from you any longer than necessary.

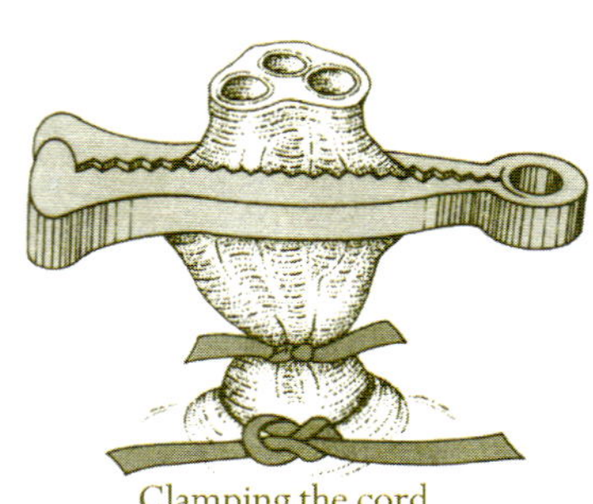
Clamping the cord

Your baby will be quite wet and messy, with some of your blood and maybe some of the white vernix still on the skin.

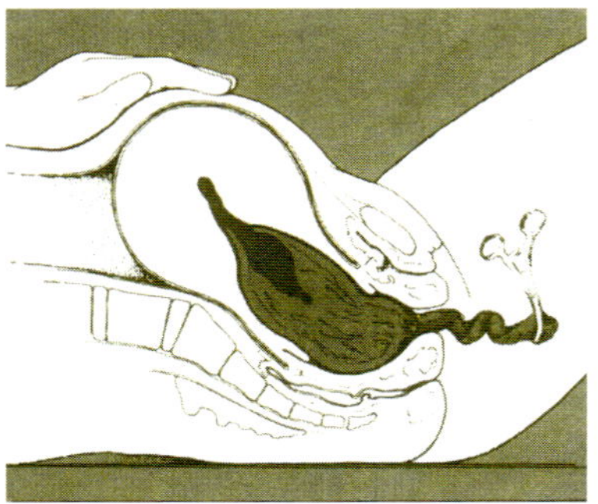
Birth of the placenta

The Third Stage
Birth of the Placenta

After your baby is born, another contraction will push out the placenta. You will probably be given an injection in your thigh just after your baby is born to help the womb to contract. You may not even notice this being done. The doctor will draw the placenta out by the cord, with maybe an extra push from you. The birth of the placenta is usually very easy.

After the birth there will be some clearing up to do. If your perineum has torn, you will be given some stitches. The nurse will wash you and freshen you up. She may clean the baby too. Your baby will be weighed and measured, and given a name band. A child specialist will examine the baby in detail and put his or her notes. Some large hospitals also take the baby's fingerprints at this stage to prevent any mix-ups.

Shortly, the baby will be with you. If you are going to breast feed, let your baby suckle as soon after birth as possible. Babies do suck this soon, although maybe just for a short time, or they may just like to feel the nipple in the mouth. It helps a lot with breast-feeding later on, and it also helps your womb to contract.

Special cases

Rhesus negative mothers

If your blood group is rhesus negative and your husband's is rhesus positive you will be given an injection (anti-D) within 72 hours of delivery in order to protect your next baby. This injection is an absolute must; without it your next pregnancy can go bad.

Induction

For most women, labour starts by itself. But for some there may be good reasons for starting labour off artificially. This is called induction. Labour may be induced if there is a risk to the baby or the mother's health—for example, if a baby is overdue, or if the mother has high blood pressure, toxaemia or diabetes. Mostly, the procedure is done in a planned way, with admission at the hospital or nursing home where your obstetrician would be in attendance.

Induction can be done by two methods. One, by breaking the bag of waters. Two, by starting the mother on an oxytocin hormone intravenous drip in the arm.

The breaking of bag of waters, called artificial rupture of membranes, soon starts off contractions if the conditions are favourable for childbirth. Thus, if the baby's head is already engaged in the pelvis, the cervix has softened and has started to dilate and pregnancy is nearer term, the outcome is usually satisfactory. The procedure however carries the risk of intra uterine infection especially if the birth does not occur within first 48 hours. There is also a very small risk of the prolapse of the baby's umbilical cord which may complicate the situation and require an emergency Caesarean section.

The second method uses oxytocin, the natural hormone which initiates the uterus into action at the time of labour and effects childbirth. It is the same hormone that is mixed in a proper dose in 5 per cent glucose solution and given in an intra venous drip to speed up the baby's birth. The method however is not always successful. Some mothers deliver with the first drip, while some may be successful with the second or third drip. If labour does not get initiated in 24 hours despite the maximum permissible dose of oxytocin, the effort is given up. If the situation is not urgent, attempts are made again a day or two later.

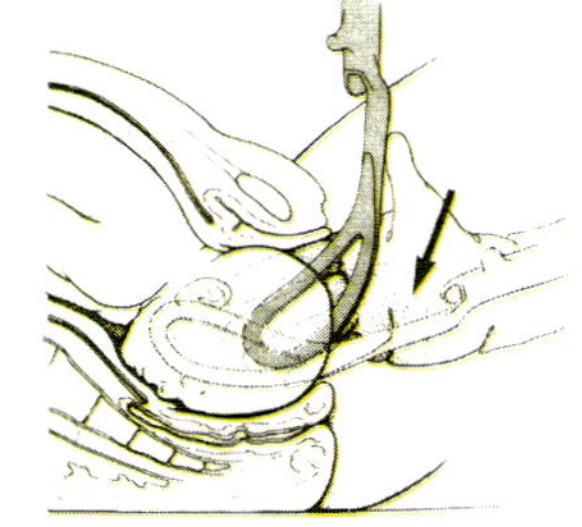

Forceps delivery

Sometimes the baby needs to be helped out of the vagina by using forceps. This is needed if the mother has become too exhausted, the uterine contractions are not strong enough, or because the baby shows signs of distress.

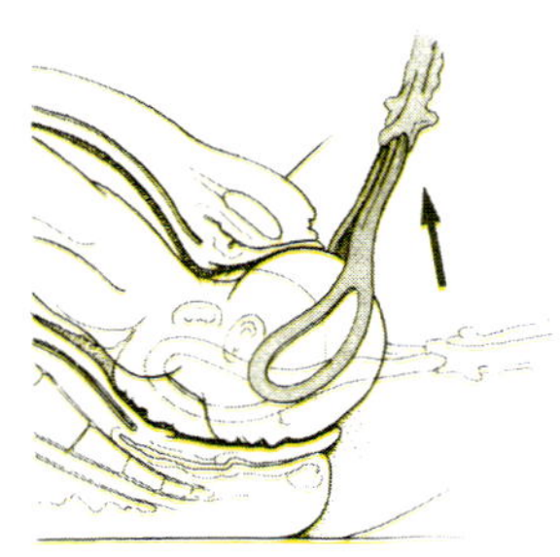

Usually a local anaesthetic is given. The forceps are placed round the baby's head and by gentle, firm pulling the baby can be born. The mother can help by pushing at the same time.

Afterwards you may find red marks on your baby's head where the forceps have been. Do not be worried; these marks would fade quite quickly.

An episiotomy (cutting the perineum to make the vaginal opening bigger) is always needed for a forceps delivery, so stitches are needed afterwards.

Vacuum extraction

This is done for the same reasons as a forceps delivery. A shallow metal cap is attached to the baby's head by suction. The baby can then be pulled out as you push. There is a swelling on the baby's head afterwards, but this gradually disappears.

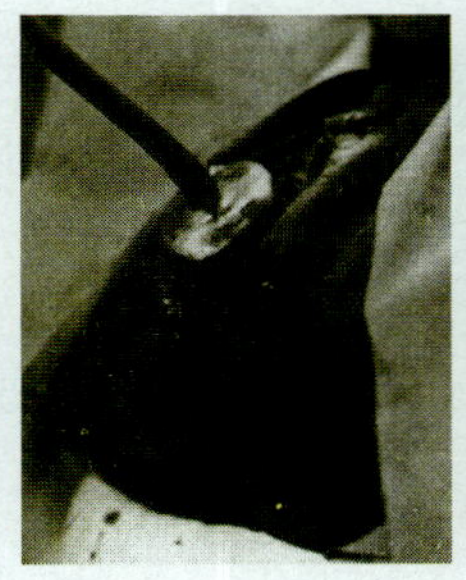

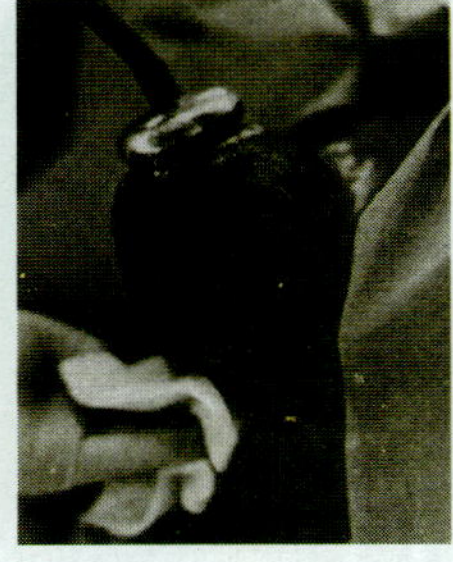

Caesarean section

Caesarean section is the surgical removal of the baby through an incision in the lower abdominal wall and the uterus. This operation has been practiced since ancient times on dead and, probably, dying mothers to save the life of the baby. According to tradition, Roman statesman Julius Caesar was born by this method, hence the name. Roman law, however, restricted the operation to women who died before childbirth, and as Caesar's mother lived long after he was born, the tradition is probably false. The first authenticated case of a Caesarean section on a living woman occurred in 1610. Because of the high mortality risk, this operation did not become widespread until the end of the 19th century, when increased use of antiseptics and advances in surgical techniques made it less dangerous.

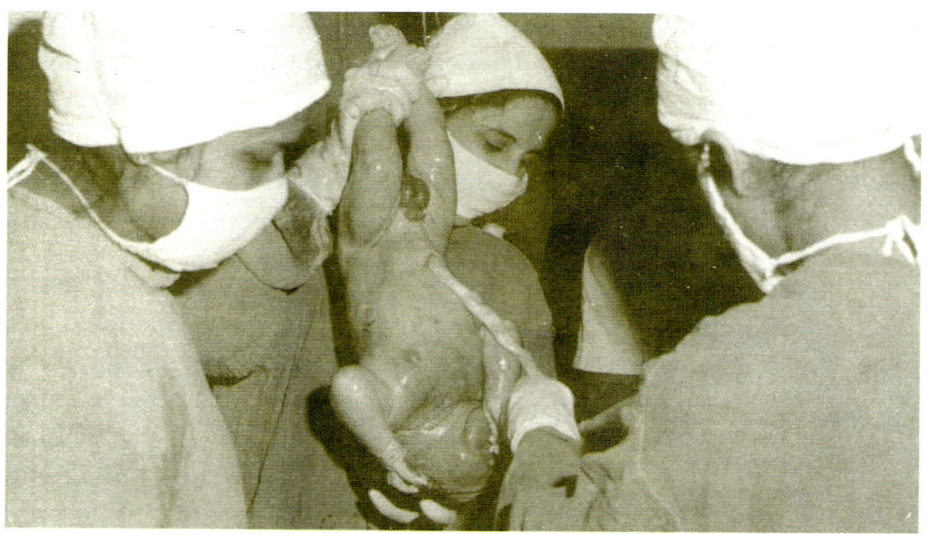

In present-day obstetrics a Caesarean section is performed for cases in which the size of the birth canal is too small to allow the baby to pass. The operation also is used in cases of abnormal developments during delivery, such as haemorrhage or tumours in the mother, failure of the cervix to dilate, baby being in distress, or difficult positioning of the baby.

The incision is usually done low down, just below the bikini line. It is hidden when your pubic hair grows again. The operation can be done under general anaesthetic or sometimes using an epidural.

With an epidural you can be awake through the operation but you won't feel pain, only some tugging and pulling. A screen will be put across you or an eye pad would be given to cover the eyes so that you cannot see what is being done. The advantage of an epidural is that you are awake at the moment of delivery, just as you would

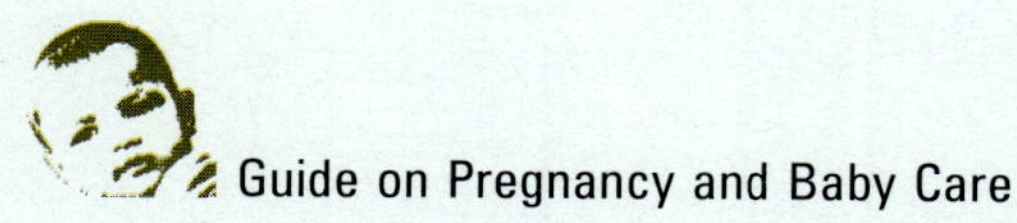

be normally, and you can see and touch your baby straightaway. It takes about 10 minutes from the start of the operation to the delivery.

After a Caesarean operation you will be uncomfortable for a few days–just as after any major surgery. It will be difficult to sit up or stand up straight, and it will hurt to laugh. You will probably have to stay in hospital a bit longer, say about a week, and it will take you rather longer to get back to normal once you are home. You must also pay sufficient attention to postnatal exercises to get your muscles working again.

Breech birth

A breech birth is when a baby is born bottom first. It is possible for a baby to be born this way quite normally but more care is needed, especially to deliver the head, so labour is usually longer. Forceps are sometimes used. A breech may be a reason for a Caesarean delivery.

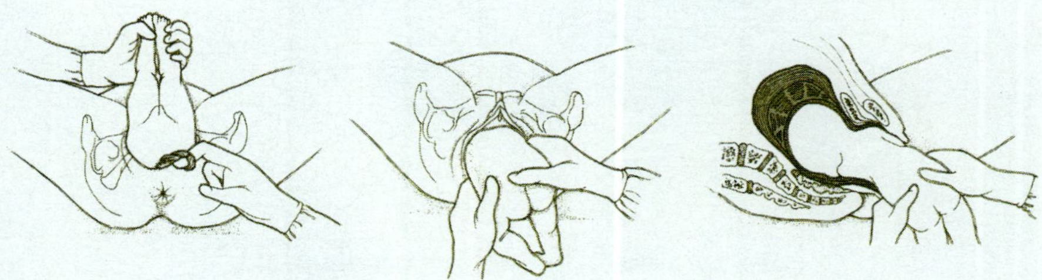

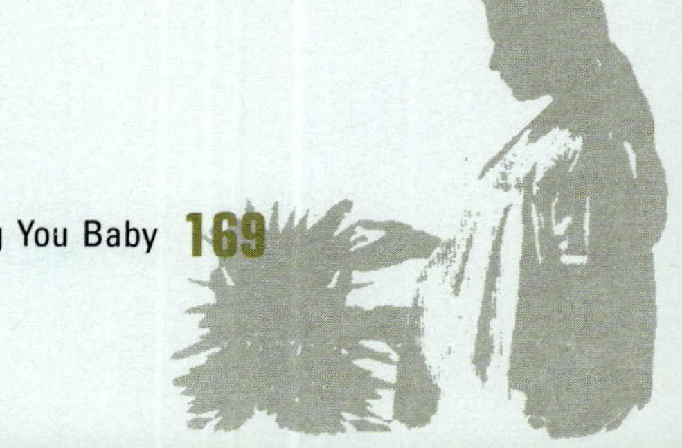

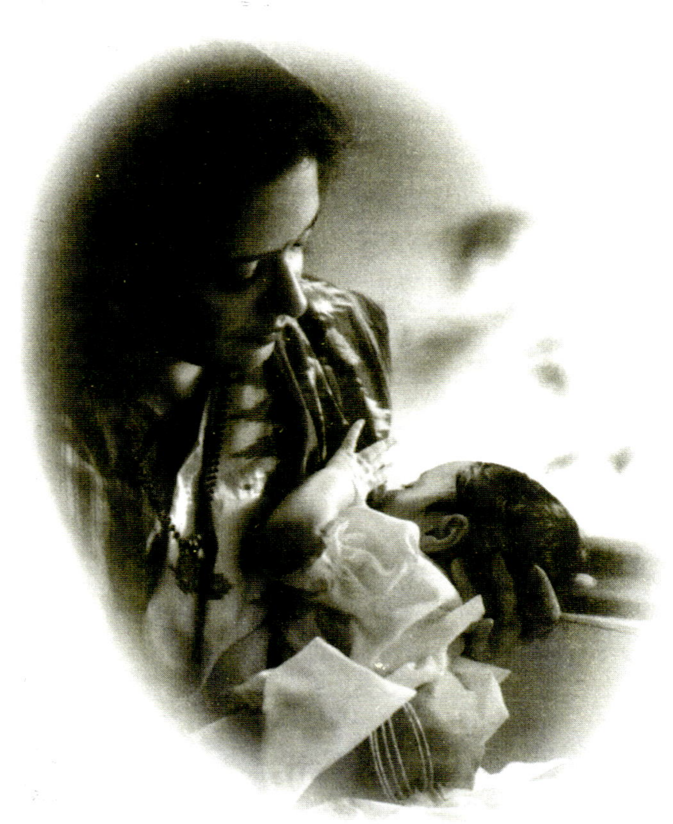

"I have no name : "I am but two days old."
What shall I call thee?
"I happy am, "Joy is my name."
Sweet joy befall thee!

-William Blake (1757-1827), English poet.
Infant Joy, stanza 1, in Songs of Innocence.

The Initial Days : You and Your Baby

Most mothers feel rather happy and contented while recovering from the rigours of childbirth. The baby offers them a medium to exalt in their new role of a mother. But, there are still a few things to cope with, and some decisions to make. For instance, the question of how soon should she be back on her feet, when to bathe, the handling of stitches, how long would the bleeding last, how to feed the baby and parenting a baby who is totally dependent on her. This takes most of her thoughts and time.

You are in a daze. Just delivered a baby some hours ago, with messages of congratulations pouring in by a dozen, discharged from the hospital, and home again with a newborn in your lap! What do you do how to cope with the advice and more advice that keeps pouring in? It is best to be sensible. Do not succumb to the myths and superstitions that your mother and her mother before her lived with and wish to percolate. Just politely accept what you know is good and healthy, and if any doubts creep in your mind, clear them by talking to your doctor or the baby's paediatrician. Give yourself time. The difficulties that crop up immediately after birth pass soon. The best is to relax and feel the pleasure of cooing to your newborn and in attending to his needs.

At the hospital

If you have had a natural delivery, most obstetricians would discharge you and the baby within the next 48 hours. Some may take a day more. But if you have had a Caesarean section, you need to stay at the hospital for about a week. Think of your hospital sojourn as a restful and easy period. You may find some things not to your liking, and that may be tiring and difficult, but it is best to adjust. Most hospitals in India work in a fashion that's very much there own, but some are more receptive. If you find you have a problem talk to the staff on the ward and see whether anything can be done. In the first few days of recuperation, it is best to limit the number of visitors. This will allow you time to rest and safeguard both you and your baby from germs that a visitor may carry to your room.

Eating

A few hours after having delivered, your appetite would return and you will feel hungry. Unless you have been given a general anaesthetic, there is no reason why you should not eat. You can enjoy a normal diet, but make sure it is nutritious and provides just the right amount of calories. Milk or milk products should be your favourite. Avoid too much of fats. Take a lot of liquids. You need them for yourself and also, to produce sufficient milk for your baby.

Getting back on your feet

In many Indian homes, the elders believe that a new mother must take complete rest during the first six weeks and at first, in the first six days, she had best not stir even out of her bed. This attitude needs a change. Even though you need an abundance of rest, and time to relax and sleep, a number of scientific studies have affirmed it is best for you to be up and about within a few hours of childbirth.

You can begin by someone assisting you in and out of your bed and walking with you as you take a few steps or walk to the bathroom. You could sit in a chair for a brief period and then increase the time gradually and on succeeding times up, increase activity gradually. This will be healthier for you. It would mean less trouble with bowel and bladder performance, and more significantly, lessen the danger of blood clots in the deep veins of the legs considerably. An early ambulation would also allow the uterus to return to its normal condition more quickly. That to why most obstetricians today encourage newly delivered mothers to be up for short periods of time beginning from the day of delivery. Even a mother who has had a Caesarean section can get up the next morning.

The older women at home may not agree to this. Your mother may nostalgically recall how she remained glued to her bed for six days (till chatti) before she could take a step, and how, for the next five weeks, she did not touch a thing, and how the rest worked wonders for her. You need not disagree wholly with her! Never let the early mobilisation to degenerate into early resumption of domestic duties and anxieties. It is best to take it easy during the first few days. In any case, with a baby to look after, you would have your hands full.

When to bathe

You can have marked perspiration in the first few days after childbirth. A daily bath, therefore, is ideal. It is both refreshing and a source of comfort. You can have a bath as soon as you start walking. Initially you should have an attendant nearby who can help you if such need arises. But if you have had a Caesarean section, just make sure that the incision is kept clean and dry.

Care of stitches

Most first-time mothers require a small incision in the perineum to enlarge the birth canal outlet. This is called an episiotomy and it facilitates an easy childbirth. The incision is closed with stitches immediately after the baby's born. You may feel a little sore for the first few days because of the stitches. It may feel difficult going to the bathroom. Even just walking and moving about can be hard work. But you can try sitting on a rubber ring for relief. It will also help to keep the stitches clean and healthy. Bathe the stitches with cotton wool and warm water mixed with dilute Savlon. After bathing, dry the area around the vagina carefully.

Going to the toilet can be difficult at first because of the soreness. If you really find it impossible to pass urine, tell the doctor or nurse.

You probably will not move your bowels for a few days after the birth, but it is important not to let yourself become constipated. Try to include some fresh fruit, vegetables or salad and roti or wholemeal bread in the food. Although it is unlikely that you will break the stitches and open up the cut or tear again, still hold a pad of clean tissue over the stitches when you try to pass a stool. And avoid straining for the first few days. These stitches do not have to be taken out. They just dissolve after a week or so, by which time the cut or tear will have closed.

Post delivery discharge

Some societies resolutely believe that the young mother is impure till she has the post-delivery vaginal discharge. In some homes, the woman is kept in a separate room as if she is an untouchable! The attitude is wrong. There is nothing unclean about either the menstrual discharge or the flow from the birth canal. Both are physiological, and should be considered so.

The post-delivery discharge continues for 10 to 14 days after the baby's birth, though it keeps changing its nature. For the first three to four days, it consists of blood, mostly fluid or containing small clots, which should not cause unnecessary alarm. It gradually becomes thinner, then brownish, and later pink and mucoid. Eventually, it loses colour and becomes white until it disappears. During this period, you must give the fullest attention to hygiene and cleanliness. Use ordinary sanitary towels, not tampons. There is a risk of infection if you use tampons in the early weeks after delivery.

Resumption of Menstrual Periods

If you are breast-feeding, you may not have another period until you stop feeding. Even then it may be some weeks or even months before you menstruate again. If you do not breast feed, you may have your first period as early as a month after delivery.

Your shape

After delivery your abdomen will be quite baggy and wrinkled. Despite losing the weight of your baby, the placenta and a lot of fluid, you will also still be bigger than you were before pregnancy. But soon you will begin to get back to your normal shape and size. Breast-feeding will help because it makes the womb contract. Postnatal exercises do one better; they help tighten the abdominal muscles and restore your looks.

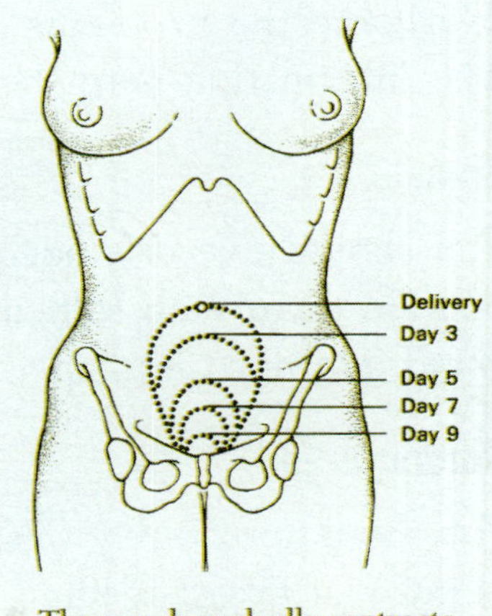

The womb gradually contracts to its normal size

The truth about witch's milk

During the first few days after birth, your breasts produce not milk but colostrum. It is a thin, yellow fluid which the elders think is unfit for the baby's consumption. You may be dissuaded from putting your newborn to the breast for the first three days. But that is all wrong. The truth is, the colostrum contains just the food your newborn baby needs and it also has antibodies, which pass on to your baby the ability to fight certain infections. By following the natural course, therefore, you do your baby a service. He would be at a lower risk of being affected by common diseases like diarrhoeas, respiratory infections and colds.

All about breast-feeding

Breast-feeding a baby is a great pleasure. If it does not go well for you at the start, do not despair and just keep working at it. Mostly, you can overcome the problems by being perseverant. The information here should help.

Breast Care

You should exercise adequate care to keep the breasts clean and provide them with sufficient support. Clean the nipples with clean water. Do not use soap.

Nursing bras

You should preferably wear a bra both day and night during the first months of breast-feeding. It will support your breasts so you feel more comfortable. A cotton bra is better than nylon one because it allows the skin to breathe. Special nursing bras are the best. They are front open and easy to remove. With normal bras, it can be very frustrating to find yourself with a hungry, crying baby and a bra that will not undo.

Your breasts and breast milk

When your milk does come in, your breasts may become very large and heavy for a while and may feel uncomfortable or even painful at first. Milk will probably leak from your nipples, but you could prevent them from getting sore by putting a clean towel to keep them dry. Gradually the amount of milk you produce will settle down and your breasts will feel normal again. So do not be discouraged by this early, rather messy and uncomfortable stage of breast-feeding.

Finding the right position

Find a comfortable position that suits both you and your baby. You have to make sure that your baby can suck easily at the breast, and that you are comfortable enough to be able to relax. Experiment to find what position works best for you. But if you would prefer to nurse the baby lying down, make sure that the baby's head is propped up. That's because babies have a very short tube between the throat and the inner part of the ear and a lying down position would allow any germs to pass into the ear, sometimes leading to a serious ear infection.

How often?

Rather than trying to stick to a timetable, it is best to feed when your baby wants to be fed. This might be very often at first. Gradually your baby will settle into a routine, probably asking to be fed every two or three hours during the first weeks. Of course, crying does not always mean hunger. It might mean a tummy ache, a dirty nappy etc. You will soon learn to know what your baby wants. And if you are not sure what is needed, it does no harm to offer a breast. Even if your baby is not hungry, sucking a little and being close to you will be comforting. A sleepy baby may need waking up to be fed.

How much?

At first it is impossible to tell how much milk your baby is taking at a feed and whether it is enough. As you get to know your baby and the feel of your breasts before and after feeds, this will no longer be a problem. Just let your baby decide how long a feed should be. The surest way of knowing whether your baby is getting enough milk is weight gain. But remember that most babies do not start gaining weight straight away, and some even lose a little early on. Your baby's weight gain will be checked each time you take him or her to the child specialist. Apart from weight, so long as your baby feeds well, and there's nothing that worries you about the contents of the nappies, you can be pretty sure that your baby is getting enough milk. A good guide to use is that a baby should feed at least six times in 24 hours. Anything less than this suggests loss of appetite.

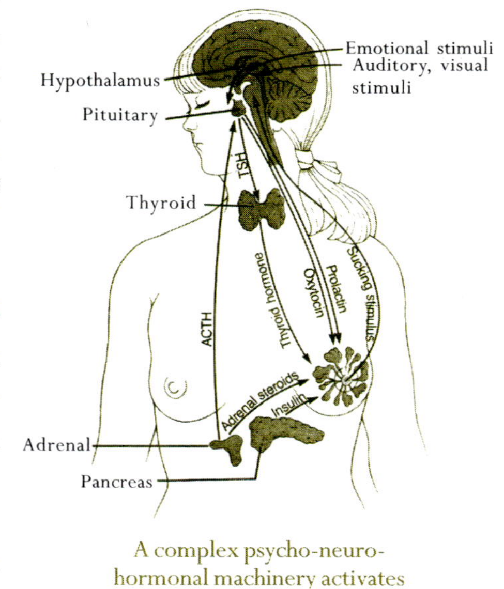

A complex psycho-neuro-hormonal machinery activates the breasts to secrete milk

How to increase the quantity of milk

At first, you may that you do not have sufficient milk for your baby. The remedy is simple: put your baby to the breast more often, and at least at every two hours. This will improve the milk let down because suckling promotes the release of the prolactin hormone in the mother. You will also benefit by taking plenty of liquids, and taking proper rest and diet.

Wind

Babies often take in air as they feed. After a feed, gentle back rubbing with your baby lying against your shoulder or held sitting upright on your lap may bring up some wind that would be uncomfortable otherwise.

Care of your baby

Babies are of all kinds, and each is so very different from the other. Some are quiet, some active and they respond in different ways to attempts to comfort and console them. A new mother must learn her baby's particular patterns and why he cries and fusses at various times. Successful mothering rests on sensible behaviour and a positive attitude.

Handling the Infant

Although they are small, newborns are not as fragile as they sometimes seem. They should he treated gently, of course, but firm, smooth handling helps them feel secure. There is no one correct way of turning, lifting, or holding a newborn, but the following points should be kept in mind:

1. The head and buttocks need to be supported.
2. Babies are wiggly and can push themselves out of your grasp.
3. It is easier to pick an infant up from the supine position than from the side-lying or prone position.

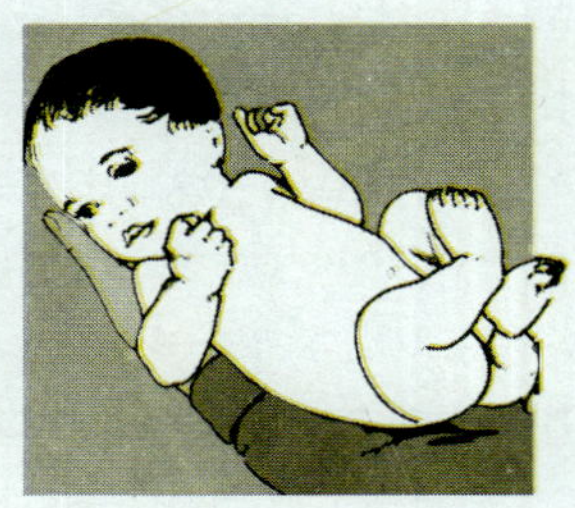

A good way to lift a baby is to place one hand under the neck to support the head and shoulders, and the other hand under the buttocks to grasp the opposite thigh. The baby can then be lifted up to a holding position or moved from one place to another. A useful position for holding or carrying is the "football hold".

Clothing the baby

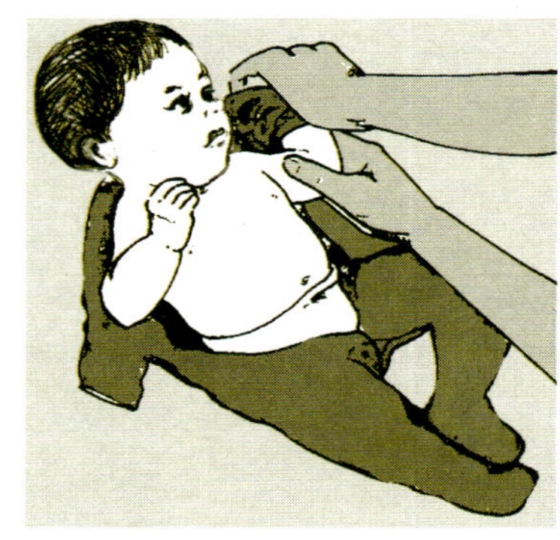

Confidence in dressing and undressing the baby comes with practice. When putting on a shirt or frock, it is helpful to reach through the sleeve with your fingers and pull the baby's hand through. Babies must be dressed suitably in keeping with the weather. If the conditions are warm, a baby needs little more than a nappy and a vest. But if it is cold, the vest must be replaced with a romper suit.

Diapering is fairly simple if you use disposable diapers that fasten with tapes. If pins are needed they should he inserted pointing toward the baby's back so there is less danger to the baby if they come open. You may also use cloth nappies (they are better than the disposable ones in many ways), and wash them after every use.

Placing the baby in the crib

You can wrap the baby snugly in a cloth before placing him or her in the crib. Some babies seem happier with their arms inside the cloth, and others like their arms free. Position the baby in the crib preferably on the side with a roll of khes or a blanket at the baby's back for support. This should extend from shoulder to hip. If it is behind the baby's head, it pushes the head forward.

Baby Facts

Soon after birth you will begin to look properly at your baby and notice every tiny detail–the shape of the hands, the length of the fingers and toes, the expressions on the face...Based on these observations some parents even begin to visualise the vocation the child would take once he grows. For instance, long fingers are taken as a sign that the child would take a creative career and would become a surgeon or an artist! But besides these interesting guesses, there may be some things you may notice and feel a little concerned about:

Soft spots in the skull

On the top of your baby's head, near the front, you will see a diamond shaped patch and another, a smaller defect, at the back where the skull bones have not yet fused together. These are called the fontanel. It will be about 12 to18 months before the bones close over them. You may notice the fontanel moving as your baby breathes. You need not worry about touching the area. There is a tough layer of membrane under the skin.

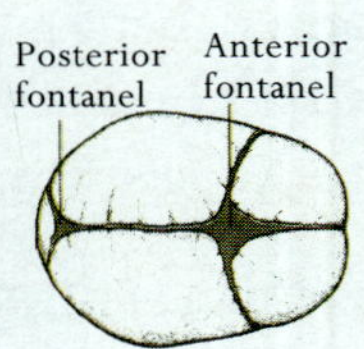

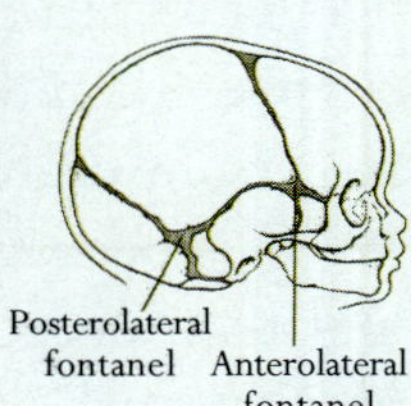

Bumps and bruises

It is quite common for a newborn baby to have some swellings and bruises on the head, and to sometimes have bloodshot eyes. The marks fade very soon.

Breasts

A newborn baby's breasts may sometimes appear a little swollen and ooze some milk on the third, fourth or fifth day. This may happen

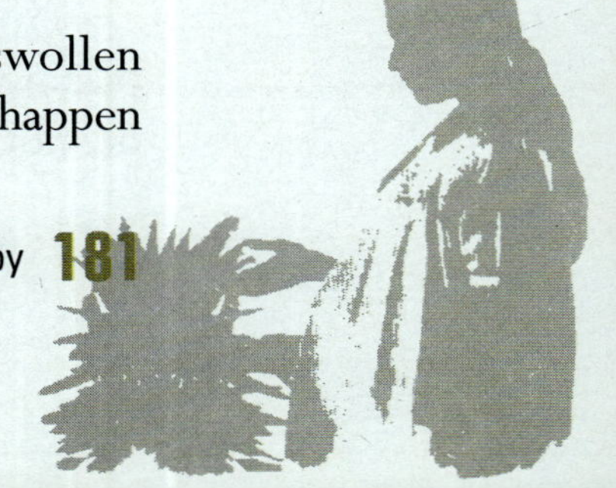

both in boys and girls. Girls also sometimes bleed a bit or have a white, cloudy discharge from the vagina between the third and seventh day. All of this is the result of hormones passing from the mother to the baby before birth. You do not need to do anything except keep your baby clean just as you would in any case.

Jaundice

After birth, some babies develop a yellow colour to their skin and yellowness in the whites of their eyes because of mild jaundice. This fades within seven days or so. But a baby who becomes badly jaundiced needs active treatment. A severe jaundice requires timely treatment and if it is caused by a mismatch of blood groups between the mother and baby, the baby will need hospitalisation and possibly, an exchange transfusion of blood. A delay in the treatment can lead to a condition called kernicterus, which causes irreparable damage to baby's brain.

Bathing and hygiene

The newborn can be given a bath from the second day. All necessary supplies should be at hand before beginning and chose an area that is free from drafts. It is preferable to employ lukewarm water (about 98°F), and wash cleanest areas first. Begin with the eyes and head and then proceed to baby's chest and back. With a little ingenuity, you can make use of equipment and facilities available at home. For instance, a large pan (parat) or basin can be used as the baby's bathtub in the early weeks. Just make sure it is kept only for the baby's use. You would also need a soft towel and washcloth, and mild baby soap. Once the cord stump has fallen off and the area has healed, you can give the baby a tub bath.

You can formulate your own routine depending on your baby's preferences. Some babies enjoy the bath as a daily routine, but others do not.

Care of Specific Areas

Eyes. The eyes should be wiped from the inner corner to the outer corner, using a clean cotton ball or clean area of the washcloth for each eye. No care, other than this cleansing with clean water, is necessary unless there is evidence of inflammation or infection. Do not use kajal or surma, because in doing so you could introduce infection into the eye. If you notice any redness, swelling, or discharge, check with your doctor. It could indicate infection.

Nose and Ears. Cotton-tipped applicators should not be used to clean the baby's nose or ears because of danger of injuring the delicate tissues. The nose usually does not need cleaning because the baby sneezes to clear the nasal passages. If some dried mucus does need to be removed from the nose, a small twisted piece of cotton moistened with water may be used. Only the outer ear should be cleaned. Nothing should be put inside the ear.

Hair. The head should be washed each time the baby is bathed. Swaddling the baby in a towel and using the "football" hold makes the job easier. The same soap the baby is washed with or any brand of baby shampoo can be used. Oil should not be put on the hair, as it may predispose to "cradle cap."

Skin. The newborn's skin is often dry and peeling within a few days after birth, and dry cracks may appear in the wrist and ankle areas. This is sometimes a cause of concern to mothers and they want to put oil or some other preparation on the skin to get rid of the dryness. You can be reassured that the flakiness and cracks will disappear in a few days and that oil and some lotions may make matters worse by causing a rash.

The sweat glands of a newborn baby do not start functioning until after the first month. The baby must always therefore be protected against warm weather and excessive clothing. Hot conditions can lead to his developing prickly heat, a closely grouped pinhead-sized rash, on the face, the neck, and wherever skin surfaces touch. Fewer clothes and a cooler clime help to relieve the discomfort.

Buttocks. Sometimes, the baby's buttocks become reddened and sore. A diaper rash can occur from a reaction of bacteria with the urea in the baby's urine. This in turn causes dermatitis. The most important prophylaxis is to keep the diaper area clean and dry. Do not be lax in changing a soiled or wet diaper. You could also use baby oil to protect the area. Pastes may not be advised, because they are much more adhesive than ointments and thus create cleansing problems. You could also expose the baby's reddened buttocks to air and light several times a day, taking care to keep the infant covered otherwise. This simple treatment is often effective. Boiling the diapers is another effective measure, since this destroys the bacteria. After washing the diapers with a detergent, care should be taken to rinse them thoroughly, since the residue of the detergent in itself can be irritating.

Nappies

It is best to use cotton diapers. They can be washed with a simple detergent or soap and reused. In contrast, disposable nappies are more convenient but expensive. In general, it is best to use them during an outing or occasionally at night. Your baby is at a higher risk of developing a nappy rash with disposable nappies, because they tend to trap the heat and humidity.

Changing nappies

1. Take off the dirty nappy and wipe away the worst of the mess with a tissue or cotton wool.

2. Clean the genitals and bottom with cotton wool and warm water, or baby lotion, or oil. Clean gently but very thoroughly. For girls, clean the bottom by wiping from front to back, away from the vagina, so that germs will not infect the vagina or bladder. Some times it may be easier to actually bathe your baby's lower half to clean more quickly and thoroughly.
3. Fold the nappy and tie on. You may like to keep some nappies ready.
4. Wash your hands thoroughly and with soap.

Cleaning and sterilising nappies

1. Flush the solid contents of the nappy down the lavatory. Sluice off the nappy, if it is soiled, in the flushing water.
2. Have ready a plastic bucket (with a lid) filled with water and the right amount of detergent powder or liquid. To make this up,follow the directions on the pack.
3. Put the dirty nappy to soak in the bucket.
4. Wash each day's nappies in very hot water. Do not use enzyme washing powders because these can irritate baby's skin. Rinse thoroughly. If you want to use fabric conditioner to soften the nappies, do not use it every time. Watch your baby's skin for any reaction.

Nappy rash

Most babies get soreness and nappy rash at some time. You will notice redness and maybe a rash. When this happens, pay extra attention to cleaning at every nappy change, and change nappies more often. It also helps to let your baby be without a nappy for a while. Even after a baby has been lying open to the air for five minutes or so, you can see the redness going down. But if the rash is severe and spreads to the thighs, it may indicate a fungal infection. This will require treatment with an anti-fungal cream, like clotrimazole. The easiest way to avoid a rash is to keep the nappy area clean and dry.

Care of baby's navel

Shortly after birth the doctor will clamp the umbilical cord close to your baby's navel with a plastic clip. She then cuts it, leaving a small bit of cord which will gradually dry out. The clamp is removed when the umbilical stump has dried sufficiently. This is usually in about 24 hours, but it might take more time for a cord that is cut long.

Care of the umbilical area usually consists of cleaning around the junction between the cord stump and the skin with alcohol to encourage drying and discourage the possibility of infection. In some hospital settings, an antibiotic ointment is used instead of alcohol. To further promote drying of the cord, the baby should not receive a tub bath until the cord has separated, and the umbilicus has healed. A cord dressing is considered to be unnecessary since exposure to the air enhances drying of the cord. No attempt should be made to dislodge the cord before it separates completely. If there is a red inflamed area around the stump or any discharge with an odour, bring it to the attention of the doctor immediately.

The cord usually becomes detached from the body between the fifth and the eighth day after birth, but it may not detach until the 12th or the 14th day. When the cord drops off, the umbilicus is depressed somewhat and usually free from any evidence of inflammation. No further treatment is necessary, except to keep the part clean and dry.

Keeping A Record Of Baby's Weight

The baby should be weighed after delivery and then every time you take him to the doctor. During the first few days after birth he may lose five to 10 per cent of his birth weight. This is due partly to the minimal intake of nutrients and fluid and partly to the loss of excess fluid. About the time the meconium (dark green faecal matter) begins to disappear from his stools, the weight begins to increase, and in normal cases does so regularly until about the 10th day of life, when it may equal the birth weight. But some babies regain their birth weight more quickly.

Sleep Pattern

The newborn needs rest and sleep, with as little handling as possible. If he is well and comfortable, he usually sleeps much of the time and wakes and cries when he is hungry or uncomfortable. He may sleep as much as 20 hours out of 24 hours! It is not the sound sleep of the adult; rather, he moves a good deal, stretches, and at intervals awakens momentarily. Since he responds so readily to external stimuli and which may make him restless, his clothing and coverings are important. They should be light in weight, warm but not too warm, and free from wrinkles. His position should be changed frequently when he is awake. He can be placed on either side or his abdomen, especially when he is ready for sleep. If he is positioned on his back, someone should be present, for if the baby regurgitates, he is more likely to aspirate in this position. As he gets older and learns to roll over, he will assume the position that he likes most for sleep.

Crying

After the baby is dressed and placed in a warm crib he usually does not cry unless he is wet, hungry, ill, uncomfortable for some reason, or is moved. One learns to distinguish an infants condition and needs from the character of his cry, which may be described as follows:

- A fretful, hungry cry, with fingers in the mouth and flexed, tense extremities, is easily recognised.
- A fretful cry, if due to indigestion, is accompanied by green stools and passing of gas.
- A whining cry is noticed when the baby is ill, premature, or very frail.
- A loud, insistent cry with drawing up and kicking of the legs usually denotes colicky pain.
- A peculiar, shrill, sharp-sounding cry suggests injury, and it is best to see a doctor.

Every effort should be made to recognise any deviation from the usual manner in which a baby announces his normal requirements. The newborn has only his posture and his voice at this time to inform others of his needs, and it is essential that the mother learn to interpret her baby's cues.

Passing urine

Within the womb, the baby's urinary activity is evidenced by the presence of urine in the amniotic fluid. The baby usually voids during delivery or immediately after birth, but the function may be suppressed for several hours. However, if the baby does not void within 24 hours, the condition should be reported to the doctor. He may need to check the baby for an obstruction in his lower urinary tract. After the first two or three days the baby voids from 10 to 15 times a day.

Stools

During foetal life the content of the intestines is made up of greenish black tar-like material called meconium. It is composed mainly of waste cells and lanugo hair that probably were swallowed with the amniotic fluid. The colour of the meconium is due to the bile pigment. Before birth and for the first few hours after birth, the intestinal contents are sterile. Apparently, there is no peristalsis until after birth, because normally there is no discoloration of the amniotic fluid.

The newborn infant passes meconium stools for the first day or two of life. After this, the stools gradually begin to change to greenish brown and then to yellowish brown. These transitional stools are less sticky than meconium and contain some milk curds. Little later, the stools take different characteristics depending on whether the infant is fed breast-milk or formula. The stools of the breast-fed infant tend to be a golden yellow colour with a distinctive odour, sometimes described as "sweet." Their consistency varies from loose to mushy, and they may be frequent or infrequent. If the infant is formula-fed the stools may be pale yellow to light brown, of firmer consistence, and may have a slightly offensive or foul odour.

Most newborns pass the first stool within 12 hours of birth; and nearly all have a stool in 24 hours. If an infant has not passed a stool by this time, conditions such as imperforate anus or intestinal obstruction must be considered as a possible reason for the delay and the baby must be observed closely.

The daily number of stools on about the fifth day of life is usually four to six. As the infant grows, this number decreases to one or two each day. The type of stool of the breast-fed baby may be influenced by the mother's diet. However, there may be slight variations from the normal, which may have little significance if the baby appears to be comfortable and sleeps and nurses well. If the baby's stools have a watery consistency, are of a green colour, contain much mucus, and flatus is being passed, it is best to check with a child specialist.

What a newborn baby can do

A newborn baby's actions are mostly reflex actions. Newborn infants can suck and swallow, move their arms and legs, and cry to make their needs known. When lying in bed, they often curl up in a position like the one they had in the womb. If startled by a loud noise or sudden jolt, they jerk their arms and legs in a reflex action called the startle reflex. Over the first few days, they very quickly learn to co-ordinate their sucking, swallowing and breathing. They also automatically turn towards a nipple or teat if it is brushed against one cheek, and their mouths open if their upper lip is stroked. Newborn babies can also grasp things, like a finger, with either hands or feet, and will make stepping movements if they are held upright on a flat surface. All these automatic responses, except of course sucking, are lost within a few months and your baby will begin to make controlled movements instead.

Development of the senses

Newborn babies can also use all their senses. The senses are known to be functional by 25 weeks gestation. In fact, some studies suggest that babies are capable of detecting changes in the intrauterine environment after 17 weeks of gestation. Mothers commonly report that the baby kicks more when music is played or quiets down when she starts rocking. Bright lights and sounds induce specific heart rate changes in the baby as he becomes aware of their presence. It is evident that the newborn is capable of perceiving environmental events at birth. The senses may be exquisitely sensitive at birth as in the olfactory sense, or they may be relatively immature as in the visual and auditory senses; however, even the immature senses perform well

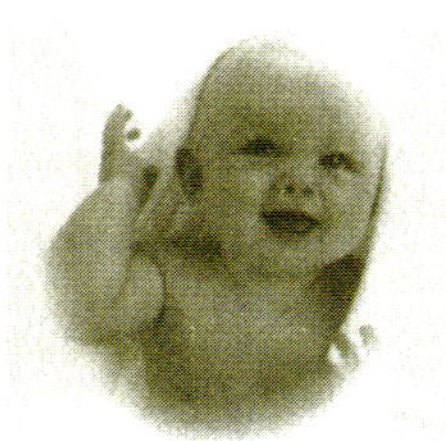

within their limitations. The full-term newborn is able to look at people and things, especially if they are near, and particularly at people's faces but he cannot control the movements of his eyes. He can hear well and will react to bright light and noise and will listen to your voice. Very soon he will learn to recognise his mother's special smell and respond to very light touch and movement.

Immunisation at birth

Babies are given the following vaccines at birth. These vaccines are safe and without any immediate reaction. Some doctors prefer to administer the vaccines a bit later. This is perfectly acceptable.
The vaccines given at birth are:

☹BCG ☹ Oral Polio ☹Hepatitis B

Registering the birth

The Central Births Act, promulgated in 1969 by the Government of India, makes it mandatory for you to register the birth within 14 days from the birth date. If the baby is born at a hospital or nursing home, the responsibility of reporting the birth falls on them. The live birth report (giving the details of birth) given to you at the time of discharge from the hospital needs to be taken to your local municipal Birth Registration Office. The Registrar will give you a birth certificate. This certificate will be required at the time of applying for school admission, making addition to the ration card and also for variety of other things such as when applying for passport of the child.

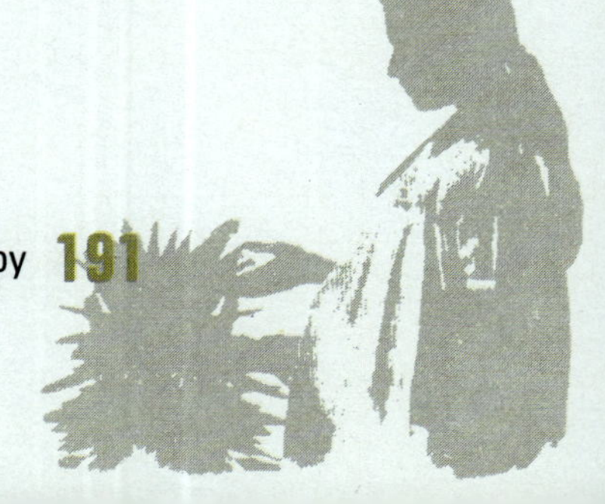

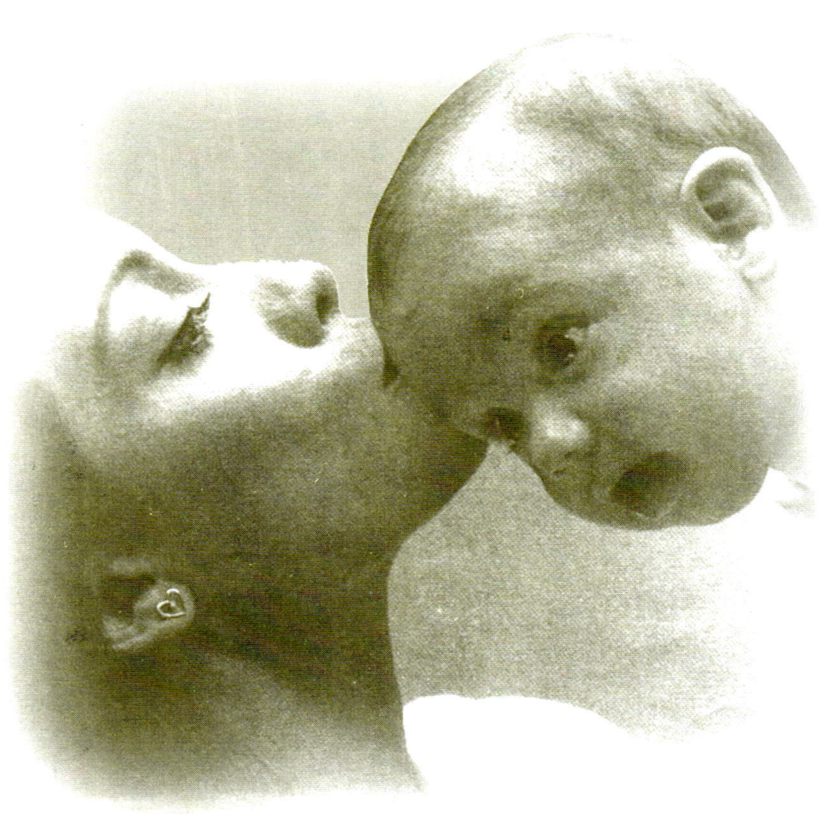

"Women know The way to rear up children (to be just),
They know a simple, merry, tender knack
Of tying sashes, fitting baby-shoes,
And stringing pretty words that make no sense,
And kissing full sense into empty words."

-Elizabeth Barrett Browning (1806-61), English poet. Aurora Leigh.

The First Year: You and Your Baby

You are exultant to be back home. The baby is in your arms and you are full of relief and excitement all at once. But you have a job still. You need to look after the baby and, at the same time, recover well from the effects of pregnancy and childbirth. There is so much to do and know before you truly begin to enjoy your new avatar. Read on for some handy advice that will hold you in good stead while your baby grows by the day and fills you with joy.

Coping with new responsibilities

Going home from hospital can be a great excitement–or just a great relief. But once you are at home, you have got quite a lot to cope with. For the first time you are looking after your baby on your own. Or, if this is not your first baby, you are coping with the demands of a number of children all at once. There are other jobs to do, like the cooking and washing. And on top of all this you may have relatives and friends visiting you. You have got to find a new routine and work out how to get things done.

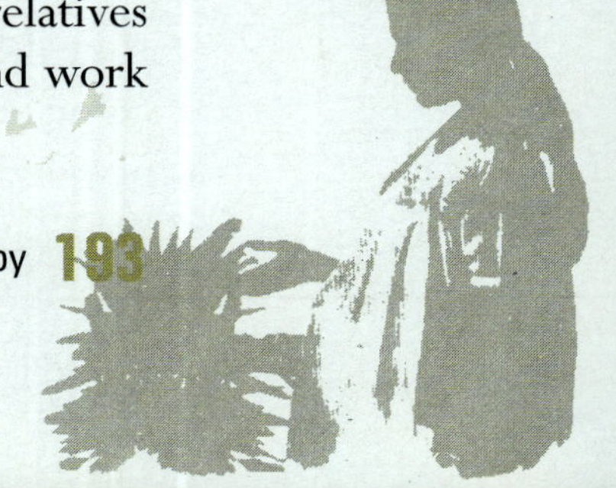

Take it easy and do not work too hard. Try and get some help. If you cannot, keep things simple so that you do not have to work all the time. For instance, if you must cook, keep your meals as simple as you can. Cut down on cleaning. And if visitors come, do not feel you have to tidy up or lay on a spread. Most of all, accept all the help that is offered. That will make life easier, and if you need it, ask for it.

You could certainly do with somebody around at first, not just to provide an extra pair of hands but also to give you support. However happy and fit you are, this can be an emotional time and it is good to have someone on hand to share problems and feelings with. For most women the best person is their mother, sister or a friend. And it is perhaps for this reason, that in traditional homes, most daughters still go back to their parents' home for confinement. But in present time, this is not always possible.

With paternity leave now becoming a rule, many fathers manage to be at home, at least, for sometime. This means they can begin to get to know their baby as well as share the work.

Relax and rest as much as you can. At a time when you are probably up at night to feed the baby and when your body is recovering after childbirth, rest is essential. At least once each day, try to sleep while your baby is sleeping, or at least put your feet up for a while. It is tempting to use the time to catch up on all the things you have not managed to do. If you have another child, choose a quiet time each day, when you can do something, like reading a story together.

What to eat

A healthy diet is very important. A good diet is what will keep you going, However tied you feel, find time to eat proper meals. They need not be elaborate. Simple dal, roti and sabji, or grilled meat or fish with vegetables or a salad followed by fresh fruit are the sort of meals that are quick to make. Do not try to reduce taste. Eat a well-balanced diet, only cut down the amount of sugar and fat intake. Have foods that are high in fibre–wholemeal bread, cereals, potatoes, fresh fruit and vegetables. These foods will prevent constipation.The fresh fruits and vegetables will also give you the vitamins and minerals you need.

Nursing mothers need an extra 550 calories each day during the first six months of breast-feeding. Later, between six months to one year, this requirement drops to 400 calories. Cheese, wholemeal bread and fruits are better choices for fulfilling this extra requirement. Breast-feeding can also make you feel more thirsty. Increase on the amount of water you drink. Also remember to avoid medicines while breast-feeding. If you need a medicine, first check on its safety. A large number of medicines are secreted in the mother's milk and can harm the baby.

Why mother's milk is best?

Breast-feeding is certainly best for your baby. It has several unmatched qualities. It is absolutely safe for the baby because it can never get contaminated with unfriendly bacteria and other germs. Rather, it confers on the baby immunity against certain infections like cough, cold and chest infections. It is the most balanced food for your baby and it contains everything a baby needs. The baby can digest it easily and is not likely to suffer from tummy upsets. Studies suggest that breast-fed babies are less likely to get fat. They just take as much milk as they need. They are also less likely to suffer from allergies like asthma and eczema. What's more, breast-feeding builds a special bond of closeness between the baby and mother and gives the baby emotional security.

Problems with breast-feeding

While at the hospital, you could always ask your doctor or the nurse to help you with any feeding problems. They can guide you on all things, no matter how small or big. When you get home, rely on any elder person or experienced mothers to help you with any difficulties. But if the problem persists seek the help of your doctor.

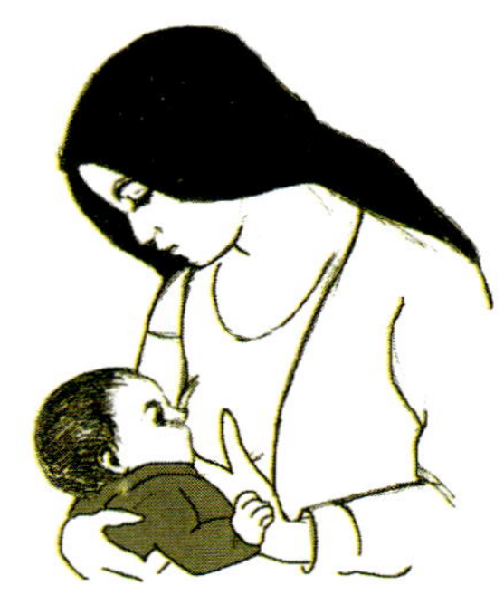

Engorged breasts

Engorged breasts are swollen with milk and by an increase in the blood supply. They may be painful and sometimes the nipple becomes flattened because of the swelling. The swelling occurs most often in the first week, starting about the time the milk discharges from the breasts. Feeding your baby is the obvious answer to the problem. If your baby can feed well, your breasts will soon improve. If a flattened nipple, or any other problem, is making feeding difficult ask your doctor for help. Sometimes the swelling and fullness does prevent a baby from being fed well. Ice packs, or bathing with warm water is helpful. Wearing a proper size brassiere will make you feel more comfortable.

Flat or turned in nipples

Flat nipples or inverted nipples are a problem simply because there is nothing for your baby to give onto. You could wear breast shells inside your bra. These may draw out the nipples. But the sucking of your baby will help the most. To facilitate this, you may use nipple shields.

Sore nipples

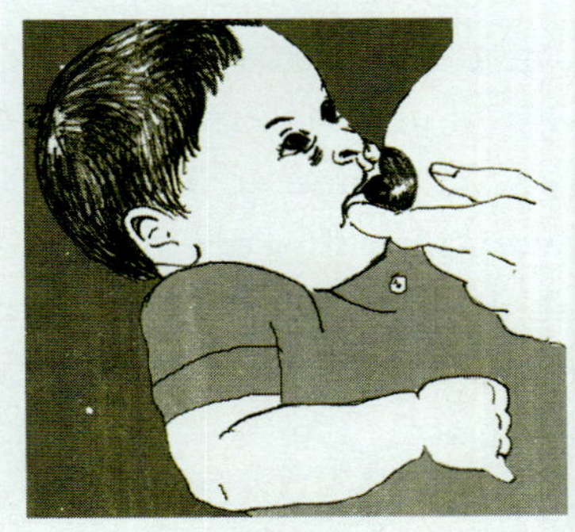

Sore nipples are quite common in the initial weeks of breast-feeding. Most often, they are the result of feeding in the wrong position. When you start to feed, hold your baby close. It may help if you hold your baby on a pillow. Touch your baby's mouth with your nipple and when the mouth is wide open, move your baby towards your breast. Aim your baby's bottom lip towards the edge of the areola, or even lower if your areola is small. Once your baby is latched on like this, feeding will not hurt, even if you are sore. Nipple shields can also give temporary relief. They are like teats which fit over your nipple, so that your baby can suck, but not on the nipple itself.

Cracked nipples

Cracked nipples are very painful. Again, make sure that your baby is feeding in the right position. As with sore nipples, correcting the baby's position will help the nipple to heal quickly.

Blocked ducts

Blocked ducts make your breast feel lumpy and tender where the blockage is. Start with the blocked breast for a couple of feeds until the blockage clears. While your baby is sucking, gently stroke over the lumpy area with your fingertips, smoothing the milk towards the nipple.

If the blockage does not clear and the skin becomes red and hot, see your doctor right away. It may be that you have mastitis, an inflammation of the breast, which needs immediate treatment.

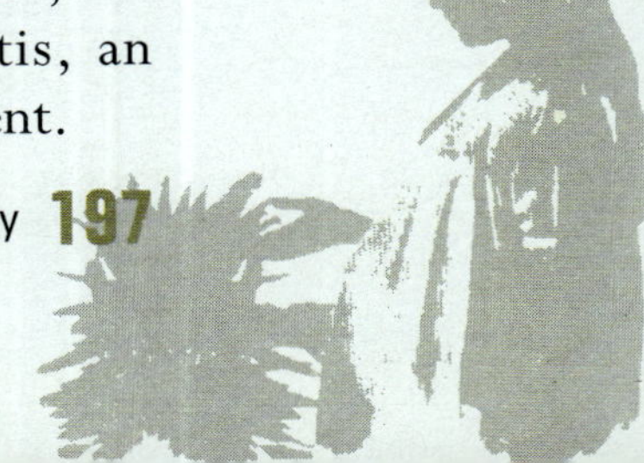

Exercise to get back in shape

Getting back into shape is every young mother's desire. The only way to fulfil this is to do postnatal exercises. Exercises not only help you to get back in shape but also make you active and fitter. It is also very common to lose control over bladder, exercises can help you overcome this problem. You must exercise regularly and not give up soon. Exercise when done regularly help you to move about more easily, regain your shape and your muscles will tighten up again. It will tone your stomach and pelvic muscles and relieve excess flab.

If not attended to, a sagging pelvic apparatus can distort the anatomy of this sensitive region. Some women even lose control over their urinary bladder. A simple forceful action such as a sneeze or a sudden cough can make them wet. Unless checked on time and suitable repair done, the womb may soon bulge from the vaginal opening. This 'prolapse' of pelvic structures can mess up middle age. It can be very troublesome, it may cause damage to the womb and certainly rob the woman of joys of sex. The only way to set it right is a major surgery. You must clearly. therefore, work at prevention.

When to start

In an uncomplicated delivery, simple exercises can be started during the first postpartum week. If the woman has had an abnormal delivery or extensive perineum repair, they can be started a little latter when the healing of the tissues is complete.

Draw a programme

The exercise programme should progress in phases, beginning with simple exercises and progressing gradually to more strenuous ones. When you are able to comfortably accomplish the repetitions of one phase, you are ready to progress to the next. You should not hurry and progress through all exercises at your own pace. As with antepartum exercises, avoid fatigue and do not do any exercises that cause pain. If the exercises are practiced properly, they should not be tiring. They should be done slowly and rhythmically, only a few times at first and gradually increased. The postural reflex needs to be re-established postpartum so that you do not continue the stance you had during pregnancy. This means you must consciously contract the abdominal and pelvic floor muscles in order to balance the pelvis again after the sudden loss of its load. Because of the hormones of pregnancy the joints are still at risk for a few weeks and good body mechanics are essential to protect the joints and ligaments. The abdominal muscles are obviously in need of an exercise. The goal is to achieve a flat abdomen and good posture, with the pelvis tilted back to realign correctly with the spine. It is not uncommon for the longitudinal muscles (recti) of the abdomen to separate during pregnancy, labour or delivery. The gaping can be slight or severe. If these muscles are not corrected, the abdominal wall will remain weakened and will not be supportive for a subsequent pregnancy. Because the recti muscles are important in controlling the tilt of the pelvis, their weakness can give rise to poor posture and pain in the lower back.

Check the anterior abdominal muscles

The following exercise may be done to see if the recti have separated. Lie on your back with knees bent. Press the fingers of one hand firmly into the area around the navel. Slowly raise your head and shoulders until the

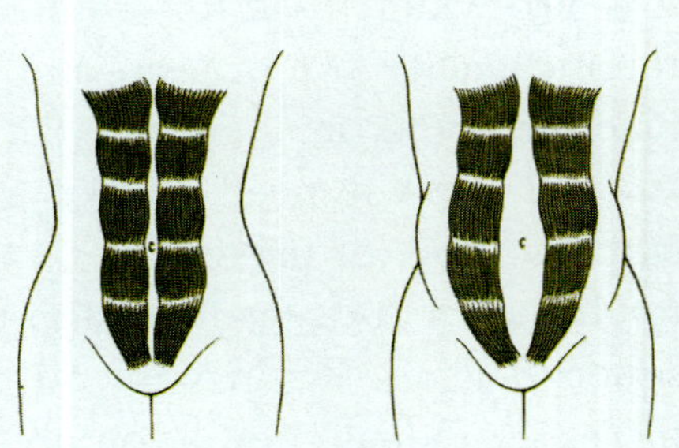

neck is about eight inches from the bed. The bands of muscles on each side will pull toward the midline, pushing the fingers out of the way. A slight gap, one or two fingers is just tissue slackness and will tighten by itself. A gap of three, four or more fingers between the muscles requires a special exercise to restore the integrity of this area.

Correct the recti before graduating to other exercises

The following exercise is done to correct the separation in the recti if it has occurred. Lie on the back with knees bent. Cross your hands over the abdominal area to pull the muscles toward the midline as head is raised. Take a deep breath. Raise the head (and later the shoulders to a 45° angle) off the bed while exhaling and at the same time pull the muscles together. Return slowly to original position. Repeat exercise often and gradually work up to at least 50 times a day. Until the separation of recti has closed, you must avoid exercises that involve rotation of the trunk, twisting of the hips or bending the trunk to one side.

Carry out Kegel's pelvic floor exercises

The purpose of the Kegel's pelvic floor exercise after delivery is to enable the muscles to resume their role in supporting pelvic contents and to re-establish sphincter control. It is an excellent exercise to maintain life-long pelvic floor tone and to enhance sexual enjoyment. It is also widely used for women with sexual dysfunction to increase their capacity for orgasm and it is helpful for minor degrees of bladder prolapse.

All that you need to do is to squeeze the muscle that is used to stop the flow of urine. This is the pubococcygeus muscle. Squeeze for three seconds (as if to stop urine), relax for three seconds, and squeeze again. Begin with 10 three-second squeezes per day and increase gradually until you are doing 25 twice daily.

You could also do the flutter exercise. Squeeze and release, then squeeze and release alternately as rapidly as you can.

You can do Kegel's exercises anywhere and anytime. Done regularly, it serves you well for the rest of your life.

Graded exercises for firming the abdomen

Phase1. Abdominal Breathing

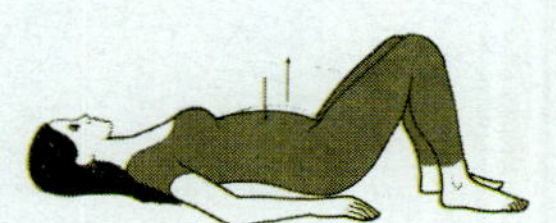

1. Lie on back with knees bent.
2. Inhale deeply through the nose, keeping ribs as stationary as possible and allowing the abdomen to expand up.
3. Exhale slowly but forcefully while contracting the abdominal muscles.
4. Hold for about three to five seconds while exhaling. Relax.
5. Begin with two repetitions, gradually progressing to 10.

Phase 2. Abdominal Breathing and Supine Pelvic Tilt

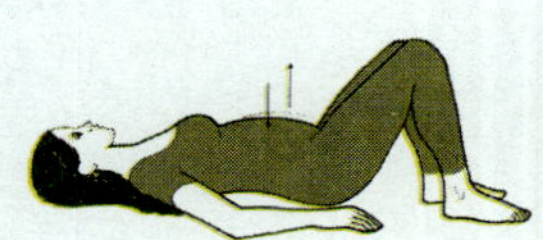

1. Lie on back with knees bent.
2. While inhaling deeply, roll pelvis back by flattening the lower back on floor or bed.
3. While exhaling slowly but forcefully, contract the abdominal muscles and tighten the buttocks.
4. Hold for about three to five seconds while exhaling. Relax.
5. Begin with two repetitions, gradually

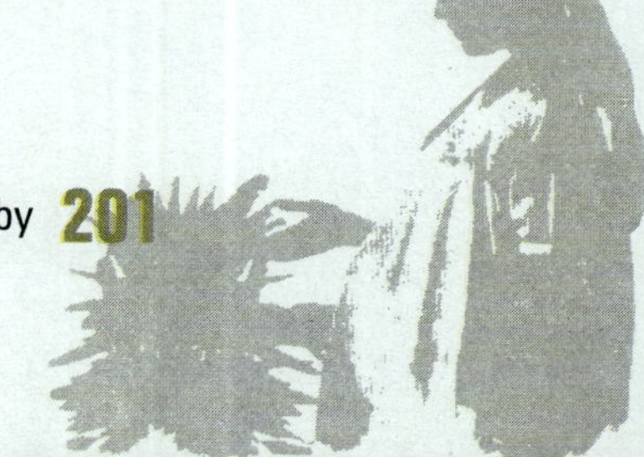

progressing to 10.

Phase 3. Reach for the knees

1. Lie on back with knees bent.
2. While inhaling deeply, bring the chin onto the chest.
3. While exhaling, raise the head and shoulders slowly and smoothly, reaching for the knees with outstretched arms. The body should only rise as far as the back while the waist remains on the floor.

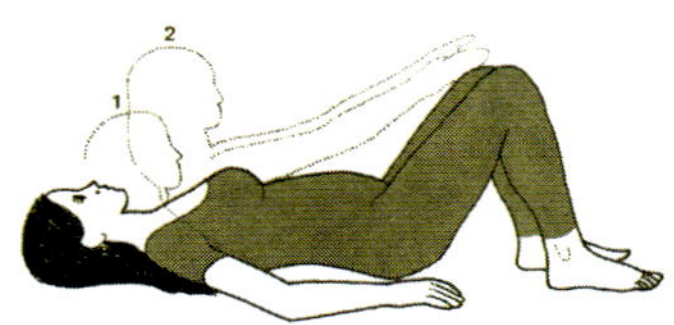

4. Slowly and smoothly lower head and shoulders to the starting position. Relax.
5. Begin with two repetitions, gradually progressing to 10.

Graded exercises for firming the waist

Phase 1. Double Knee Roll

1. Lie on back with knees bent.
2. Keeping shoulders flat and feet stationary, slowly and smoothly roll the knees over to touch the right side of the bed.

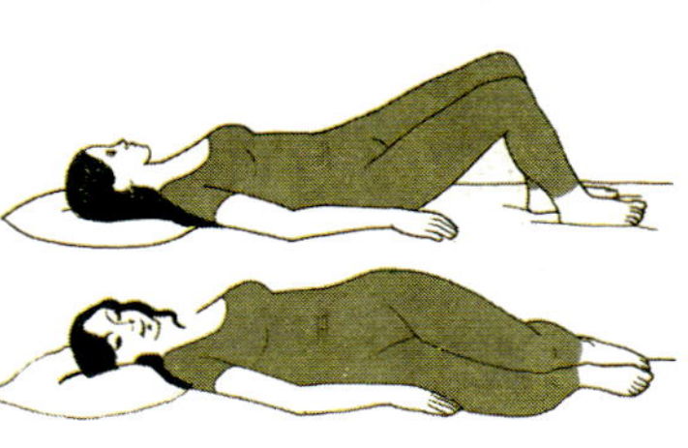

3. Maintaining a smooth motion, roll the knees back over to touch the left side of the bed.
4. Return to starting position. Relax.

5. Begin with two repetitions, gradually progressing to 10.

Phase 2. Single Knee Roll

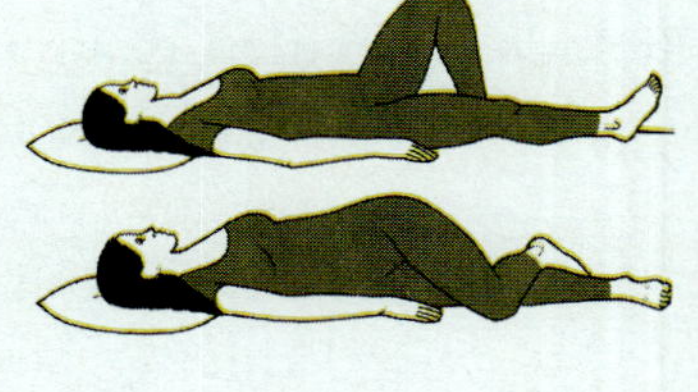

1. Lie on back, right leg straight, left leg bent at the knee.
2. Keeping the shoulders flat, slowly and smoothly roll the left knee over to touch the right side of the bed and back to starting position.
3. Reverse position of legs, touch left side of the bed with the right knee and return to the starting position.
4. Begin with two repetitions, gradually progressing to 10.

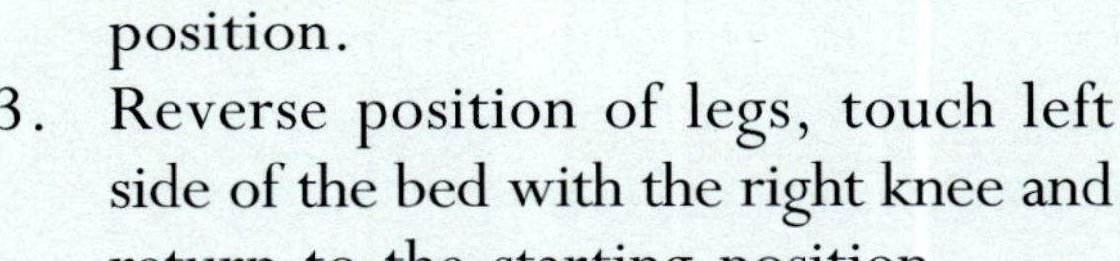

Phase 3. Leg Role

1. Lie on back with legs straight.
2. Keeping shoulders flat, slowly and smoothly lift the left leg and, keeping it straight, roll it over to touch the right side of the bed and return to the starting position.
3. Repeat, using the right leg to touch the left side of the bed. Relax.
4. Begin with two repetitions, gradually progressing to 10.

Walking is excellent

Besides these exercises, try to fit in a walk with your baby in a pram if the weather permits. It is good to get out and walking is a relaxing exercise.

Postnatal check-up

You should go back to your obstetrician for a postnatal check-up four to six weeks after your baby's birth. The check up will usually include a detailed examination:

- You will be examined to check whether your stitches (if you had any) have healed, whether your womb is returning back to its normal size and whether all the muscles you used during labour and delivery are also returning to normal.
- If you had any difficulty during the pregnancy, such as high blood pressure, anaemia, or urine infection you will be checked to ensure if all is normal now. Steps will be taken to mend the situation.
- This will also be a chance to talk to your doctor. Ask all the questions you want to. It is a good opportunity to sort out any problems or worries.

Resuming Sex

It is really for you and your spouse to decide how soon you begin to have sex again. There is no physical reason why you should not make love as soon as you feel like it. But for some weeks many couples and understandably, many women in particular feel much too tired or just do not want to have sexual intercourse. It is important to wait until you feel ready for an intercourse and when you do, to remember that it may take a while for the old responses to come back.

Contraception

If you want to space your next child, you should use contraception. It is possible you may conceive even if your menstruation is not restored. Remember that breast-feeding is not a reliable means of contraception. You will probably not start having periods again while you are feeding, but this does not mean that you cannot conceive. You can discuss the choice of contraceptive with your doctor when you visit her or him for your postnatal check-up. The possible methods of contraception are:

- The Intra Uterine Device (IUD). A copper-T inserted at the time of postnatal check-up makes a very good choice, unless your body finds it unsuitable or your doctor thinks that it would not be appropriate for you.
- The Condom. Used by the man, a lubricated sheath or a condom may be the best and simplest choice during the first few weeks. It works best if you use a spermicidal cream or jelly as well.

Copper-T

- The cap or diaphragm. A cap or diaphragm used before having a baby may not fit afterwards and so would not be reliable. You can have a new one fitted at your postnatal check-up.
- The pill. If you are not breast-feeding, you can go back to taking the contraceptive pill. But remember that it is not reliable for the first 14 days, so for this time you will need to use some other sort of contraceptive such as the sheath as well.

  If you are breast-feeding, it is best to avoid the pill though a low-dose progesterone only pill is considered safe.

Stretch marks

After your baby is born, stretch marks will gradually fade. They will never go away completely, but they will become less noticeable with time. If you wish to use oils and creams, go ahead. It is very doubtful whether they really help, but they do no harm and can be comforting. Using vitamin E creams may be most useful.

Going back to work

If you are to go back to work, you should begin to make plans well in advance. It is not always easy to find a satisfactory arrangement and it may take you some time. It is essential to feel happy and confident about whatever arrangements you make. Once you are working again, it is difficult to make new arrangements.

If your mother or mother-in-low lives with you or somewhere close by, it may be best to leave your baby with her every day. The alternative is a housemaid, if you can afford one or a crèche close to or at your place of work. A crèche can be a good solution because you can see your baby, even breast feed if you wish, in your lunch break. But unfortunately very few employers provide crèches. Day nurseries are also mostly privately run and arrangements exist for care of children of different ages. Till proper arrangements are made, it is best to extend your maternity leave.

Weaning onto a bottle

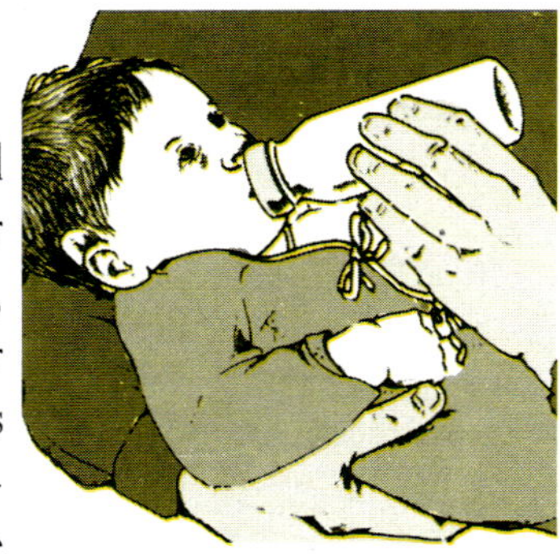

It is best to keep the baby on breast feed alone at least until the first three or four months. But if you are going back to work, then you will want your baby to switch over to the bottle. However, if you keep options open it is still possible to carry on breast-feeding, at least for sometime, after you are back from work. The changeover to formula milk should be gradual. At first change one feed each day, then another and then another. If you want you can combine breast and bottle-feeding and there is nothing wrong with it.

Bottle-feeding

Bottle-feeding may seem like hard work at first, but you will soon get into an easy routine of sterilising bottles and preparing feeds. One advantage of bottle-feeding is that fathers can participate and enjoy holding a warm and contented baby during the feed.

Cleaning and sterilising

It is important to keep every piece of your bottle-feeding equipment absolutely clean to protect your baby against infection. This means sterilising as well as washing. The best way to sterilise is to boil your equipment. You have to boil for at least 10 minutes.

Preparing the feed

When preparing feeds, mix the water and milk powder in exactly the right proportion. This is important, so read the instructions on the tin or packet carefully. Milk powder is very carefully balanced for your baby, so do not be tempted to add a little extra powder for a 'richer' feed or add any sugar. It is best to make up a bit more than your baby is likely to drink. If it is left over at the end of the feed, throw it away. The routine for preparing a feed goes like this:

- Clean your hands with soap and water.
- Boil some water and let it cool.
- Take a bottle and teat out of the vessel in which they were sterilised. Rinse them with the same water in which they were boiled. Do not rinse under the tap. If tap water gets inside the bottle or teat, it will make them unsterilised.
- Using the measuring marks on the side of the bottle, fill the bottle with the right amount of water. Use the boiled water that you left to cool.

- Measure the exact amount of powder, using the special scoop provided with the milk. Do not be tempted to pack the powder down tight.
- Add the powder to the water in the bottle.
- Screw on the cap and shake well until the powder has dissolved.

Feeding

Your baby will gradually settle into a routine, probably with feeds every three or four hours. Before you start to feed your baby, always check that the milk is not too hot by dripping some on the inside of your wrist. Babies do not mind cold milk, but they usually like it better warm. If you want to warm up the milk a little, place the bottle upright in some hot water, keeping the teat out of the water. But never keep milk warm for more than one hour. If it is kept warm for too long, harmful bacteria can grow and give your baby an upset stomach.

Choose a comfortable place and position for feeding that lets you hold and cuddle your baby comfortably. Have all the things you will need in easy reach, including a clean cloth to wipe up any spills. If there are long pauses during a feed, cover the teat with the cap to keep it clean. Never prop up the bottle and leave your baby to feed alone. It could lead to choking. After a feed, gently rub or pat your baby's back to make him burp. Your baby will enjoy being cuddled close to you after a feed.

Feeding schedules

Most babies require five or six feeds a day until they are about three months old. They can then move to taking four or five feeds daily. After they are five or six months old, most babies can go on a schedule of three meals a day with between-meal snacks.

Some common concerns about feeding

There are some areas related to baby's feeding that are of concern to the new mother regardless of the method of feeding:

Hunger

You may wonder how to know if your baby is getting enough to eat. Well, most babies when awakened from sleep by hunger pains will fuss and cry and make sucking movements with their mouths. But, if the baby awakens a short time after a feed, you should try other comfort measures such as holding, changing the diaper and bubbling, before assuming he is hungry. If he is obviously hungry and crying, seizes the nipple ravenously when a feeding is offered and nurses with great vigour, he may need to "refill" more frequently if he is breast-fed or be offered more in his bottle, at each feeding, if he is bottle-fed.

Bubbling (burping)

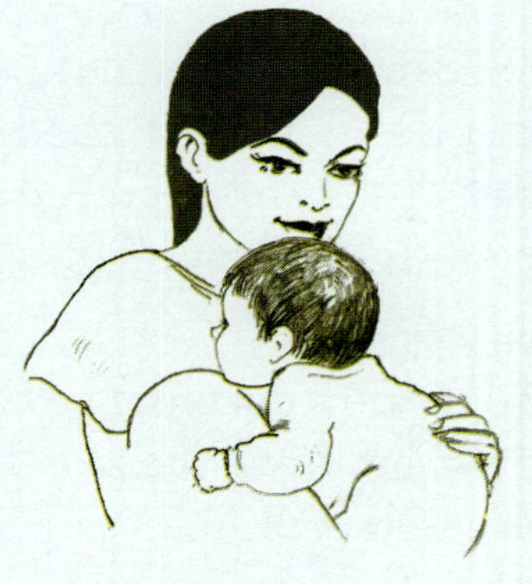

After each five minutes or so, or in the middle and at the end of each feeding, the baby should be held in an upright position and his back gently patted or stroked. The will give baby a chance to eruct the air bubbles that he would have swallowed during the feed. You should have a napkin handy to clean the mess. If there is doubt about whether or not the baby has brought up all the air, then while placing him in the crib, put him on his right side or in a prone position. This will help bring up the air. It will prevent the baby from choking on any milk that might be regurgitated with the air.

Regurgitation

Regurgitation is common in babies. It is merely an overflow of milk

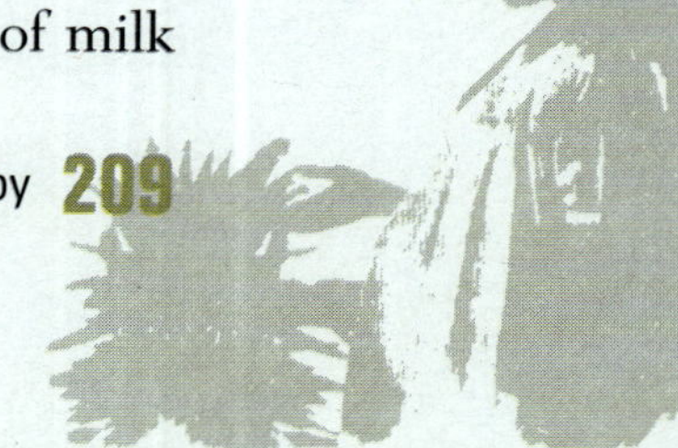

and often occurs after nursing. It should never be confused with vomiting, which may occur at any time, is accompanied by other symptoms and usually involves a more complete emptying of the stomach. This regurgitation is the means of relieving an over distended stomach. It usually indicates that the baby has taken either too much food or has taken it too rapidly.

Hiccups

Some mothers need a reassurance that hiccups are not unusual for babies and really do not seem to bother them. If the mother is disturbed, she can try giving the baby a few sips of water, but the hiccups go away by themselves without treatment.

Constipation

This is almost nonexistent in breast-fed babies and uncommon in those fed commercially prepared formulas, but mothers frequently express concern about possible constipation. Many parents believe that a baby is constipated if he misses having a bowel movement one day. That's incorrect. A baby is constipated only when the stools are hard, formed and difficult to pass.

Vitamin drops

Your baby does not need anything for the moment besides your milk, but from one month of age you may be advised to give vitamin drops as well. You can get these from the well baby clinic.

Introducing solid foods

During the first four to five months, a baby finds complete nutrition in mother's milk. But as he grows, he needs additional nutrition. One way to tell that a baby is ready for solid foods is when he appears hungry despite taking frequent breast feeds and appears to show an interest in food. In contrast, if the baby cries or turns away from such food, do not force him. Go back to breast or milk feeds for a week or two and then try again. Forcing and coaxing inevitably leads to difficulties.

It always pays to keep the environment happy and relaxed and to respect baby's appetite and food preferences. Go slow; try out one new food at a time and wait for four or five days before trying another. Watch for any allergic reaction such as diarrhoea, vomiting or rash. If these occur, stop the food and talk to your doctor.

It is best to try home-cooked fresh foods rather than tinned or bottled baby foods. The latter are convenient but expensive and are certainly not superior to homemade foods. You should avoid adding extra sugar or spices and should preferably restrict salt until eight or nine months of age.

To prevent the child from choking make him sit up when you give him food. Use a spoon and do not put solids in a bottle.

Number and Timings of Solid Feeds

At four to six months

Continue to breast- or bottle-feed four or five times a day and introduce solids twice, say around 10 am and 6 pm.

Between six and nine months

Continue to breast or bottle-feed three or four times a day and offer the baby solids three times a day, say at 9 am, 1 pm and 7 pm. You may also give him milk in a cup and stop using a bottle.

Beyond nine months

Give the child solids four times a day, say at 9 am, 1 pm, 4 pm and 8 pm. You may also give him fresh milk two or three times or continue breast-feeding.

Choice of foods

At five to six months

Mashed Fruits. Start with a quarter of a mashed banana and increase the quantity every week. Later stewed apple (peel, cut into bits, steam and mash with a spoon), papaya, chikoo, mango and pears may be given.

Vegetables. Start with a thin soup of carrots, pumpkin, doodhi, beetroot and tomatoes. Try peas, beans and leafy vegetables sometime later. Gradually you can try giving a thick soup.

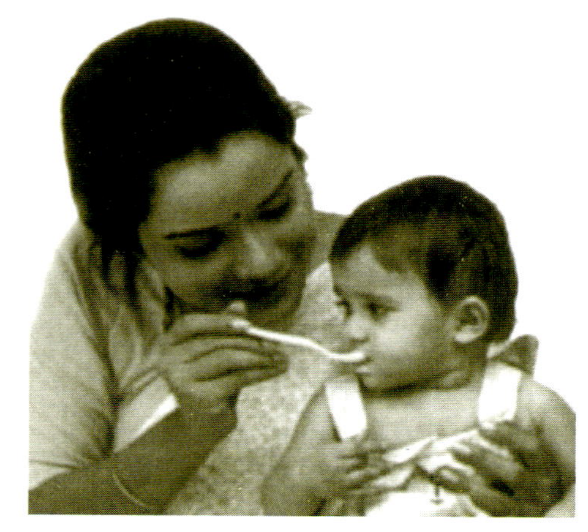

Cereals. You could begin with rice. Rice with moong dal in the form of a khichdi makes an excellent choice. Other cereals like rava kheer, thin wheat seera, dalia, sooji, ragi, biscuits soaked in milk can be tried a little later. A highly nutritious mix can be made out of roasting, grinding and mixing equal parts of rice, wheat, and ragi and moong dal. The mixed powder is stored in an airtight container. This powder can be used for making a thin kheer with milk and a bit of sugar.

Fruit Juice. Orange and apple juice may be offered like a drink between feeds.

Seven to nine months

Potatoes. You can try mashed potatoes with a bit of butter. Some babies also enjoy mashed vegetables.

Curd or yoghurt.

Eggs. Boil the egg for three minutes. Start with a quarter of the yellow part, and gradually include the white. Remember, eggs are rich in cholesterol and it is best for the baby not to have an egg more than three times a week. Some babies may also show allergy towards eggs.

Meat and other non-vegetarian foods: You can get the baby started on them.

10 -12 months

You can give the baby a normal diet. Roti, rice, dal, upma, idli, non-vegetarian foods and fruits can be offered.

Baby's Progress Card

You should take the baby to a nearby well baby clinic for follow up advice. Such clinics are run both by the government and by private practitioners. On each visit the baby will be weighed and record will be kept of the amount of weight he gains. This is one way to check that the baby is feeding well and thriving.

At most well baby clinics, adequate facilities are available for baby's immunisation and development checks and tests. The doctor will check your baby's health and progress from time to time and you can share your concerns with him.

Weight gain

During the first three months, the baby should gain between 150 to 200 gm in weight per week. From here on and till his first birthday, he should gain approximately 400 gm in weight every month. Thus, at five months of age, a baby usually doubles his birth weight, and triples it by his first birthday. This gain in weight is one good indicator of baby's health and development. If the baby is not gaining in weight or is slow to gain weight, this must be taken note of and a child specialist should be consulted.

Height increase

On an average, the baby measures 50 cm at birth; 60 cm at three months, 70 cm at nine months and 73 to 75 cm at one year of age.

Head circumference

At birth the baby's head circumference is more than his chest circumference and is about 35 cm. It increases to 40 cm by the time he is three months and is about 45 cm on his first birthday.

Chest circumference

The circumference of chest is about 3 cm less than the head circumference at birth. The two become equal by one year and from here on the chest circumference grows at a faster pace than the head circumference.

Eruption of teeth

The lower central incisors are the first teeth to appear, usually between the ages of five to eight months. The corresponding upper teeth appear about a month later and the lateral incisors (the tooth next to central incisor) usually appear within the next three months. The first molars appear around the age of 12 or 15 months.

Developmental milestones

As the baby grows, he begins to control his body better. He also goes through a socio-personal development and learns to adapt himself to the environment. This maturation of different functions (milestones) occurs at a predictable age, within the range of a few months, and is a good guide to baby's progress. Here's the road to progress:

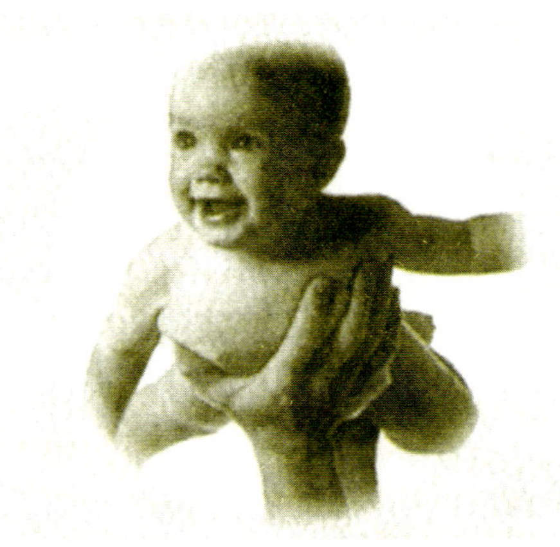

Six to eight weeks	Looks at mother and smiles.
Three months	Can hold his head erect. Recognises his mother.
Four to five months	Begins to reach out for objects. Recognises mother.
Six to eight months	Can sit without support. Experiments with noises. Can transfer objects from one hand to another. Enjoys hide and seek. Enjoys watching his image in the mirror.
Nine to10 months	Starts crawling. Can make increasing range of sounds. Releases objects. Tends to be suspicious of strangers.
10-11 months	Can stand with support. Can pull himself up from the supine to sitting position. Can creep on the floor. Begins to utter his first words.
12-14 months	Begins to walk with a wide base. Tries to feed himself with a spoon. Can build a tower of two blocks.

Immunisations

The well baby clinic doctor will also immunise your baby against certain serious illnesses. In the first year, your baby will be immunised against tuberculosis, whooping cough, diphtheria, tetanus and polio. These are all dangerous diseases and can cause permanent damage to a child's health or can even kill. Immunisation gives the child a complete protection against these diseases except in the case of tuberculosis. You may also immunise your baby against other illnesses, such as measles, mumps, rubella, hepatitis and meningitis.

Recommended Immunisation Schedule

Vaccine	Due age	Due date	Given on
BCG OPV (1) + HEP B (1)	At birth At birth		
HEP B (2)	4 weeks		
DPT (1) + OPV (2) + HIB (1)	8 weeks		
DPT (2) + OPV (3) + HIB (2)	12-14 weeks		
DPT (3) + OPV (4) + HIB (3)	18-20 weeks		
Measles + OPV + HEP B (3)	8-9 months		
Chicken Pox (optional)	12-18 months		
MMR HIB (booster)	15-18 months 15-18 months		
DPT + OPV (1st booster)	18-24 months		
Hepatitis-A vaccine (optional)	2 years		
Typhoid shot	3 years		
DPT + OPV (2nd booster) Hepatitis-A (optional) MMR (unless both Measles & MMR have been given)	5 years 5 years 5 years		
Typhoid Oral	6 years		

Typhoid Oral	9 years
Tetanus Chicken Pox Vaccine (If vaccine has not been administered earlier and there is no past history of chicken pox)	10 years 10 years
Typhoid Oral	12 years
Tetanus Toxoid (TT)	16 years

DPT	Diphtheria, Pertussis (whooping cough), Tetanus
OPV	Oral Polio vaccine
MMR	Measles, Mumps, Rubella (German measles)
BCG	Tuberculosis vaccine
HIB	Hemophilus Influenza B Vaccine (meningitis vaccine)
HEP B	Hepatitis B vaccine
Varicella Vaccine	Chicken Pox vaccine

If any of the vaccines are missed, you should talk to the doctor. Mostly, the vaccine can still be given.

Caution: Before vaccinating the child, you should inform the doctor if your child:

- Is unwell in any way
- Has ever had fits or convulsions
- Has had a reaction to the last dose
- Has a past history of any allergies
- Has any chronic or serious disease

Crying

Crying usually means that a baby is hungry, needs a clean nappy, or is uncomfortable, tired, or neglected. Once the situation is

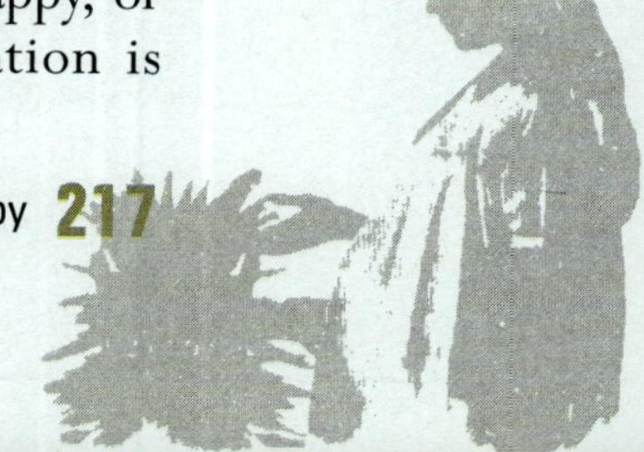

corrected, most babies ordinarily stop crying. You can also soothe the baby by offering him a "dummy" pacifier, a rubber teat attached to a plastic guard, to suck on. By now, you would understand your baby's cues rather well and know how to deal with him.

Remember, if a baby is crying he is trying to say something. He would rarely, if ever, cry without a reason. In the first months of life your baby had lived in a very comfortable, trouble-free place. Everything was made to order and all comforts were automatic! Now, afterbirth, there is a great deal to adjust to–unfamiliar sights, alien sounds and new sensations, a new way of feeding, people, clothes, nappies, baths. Perhaps crying is not so surprising. Soothing talk, singing, gentle movements like swaying or rocking, and perhaps more than anything closeness to you will all help. Sometimes babies stop crying when pushed in a pram, taken out in a car, or put into a baby carrier. You may want to try a pacifier. Many babies find a pacifier soothing. But never use a sweetened pacifier or bottle to soothe your baby. If your baby develops a taste for sweetness now, it will be difficult to break the habit later.

It can take a great deal of patience to soothe a crying baby. Often, especially if you are tired, it may need more patience than you feel you have got! But never lose your cool with the child. He cannot react to your being unreasonable.

If at any time for any reason you are worried about your baby's crying, contact your doctor. A change in a baby's crying, so that it seems different or unusual, may be the first sign of illness, particularly in a baby who is not feeding well or will not be comforted.

Sleeping Pattern

Babies sleep up to 20 hours a day during the first month after birth. Their need for sleep then gradually decreases. By about three months

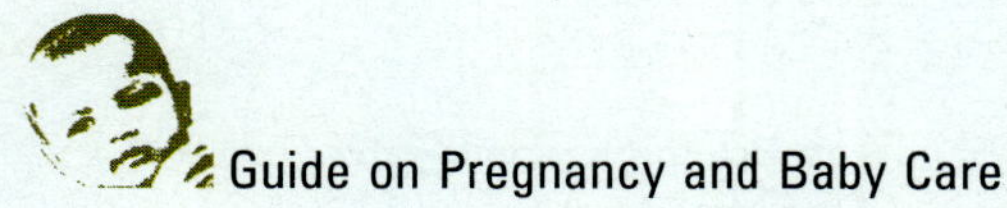

of age, most infants begin to enjoy a playful waken period each day. At such times, you may very well put the baby near other members of the family. After a play period, the baby may be fed, changed and put back in bed.

Babies sleeping patterns vary a lot. When they are very small, many babies sleep for most of the time between feeds. Others remain awake for long spells. As they grow older babies begin to develop some sort of pattern of waking and sleeping. This pattern will change as time goes by. It is unlikely to be the same pattern as that followed by other babies you know. Just as some babies cry more than others, some sleep more than others. You will gradually learn to recognise when your baby is ready for sleep and can be happily put down. A baby that is used to being put to bed when ready for sleep, but not before, is more likely to settle into an undisturbed sleep. Some babies settle better after a warm bath. Most sleep after a good feed. A baby who wants to sleep is not likely to be disturbed by ordinary household noises, so there is no need to keep the whole house quiet while your baby sleeps. It is best if a child gets used to sleeping through a certain amount of noise!

For the first two months or so, the safest way for babies to sleep is on their fronts, head to one side, or else curled up on one side. Then, if the baby vomits, there is no chance that he will choke. Babies should not use pillows because of the danger of suffocation.

Making Things Interesting . . . For Your Baby

Even very young babies like to have interesting things to look at– brightly coloured beads, for example, hung across the pram, a soft toy in the cot or a moving toy overhead.

As your baby begins to spend more time awake, you need to provide more entertainment.

Tie string across the cot, high enough to hang things from. You can then give your baby a variety of things to look at. Choose objects with contrasting colours—old greetings cards, a multi-coloured ball or toy, strips of coloured foil and so on. Change the objects every now and then and be imaginative. Some objects that make interesting, but quite gentle noises, are also good playthings such as a rattle, or a musical box. See whether your baby will turn to the noise and then follow it as you move the rattle around.

The more objects and pictures you put around your baby's cot, the more you will have to talk to your baby about. The sound of your voice is more important to your baby than any other noise, but it is not always easy to find things to chat about. Some pictures round the cot will give you plenty to talk and make up stories about.

Whatever you use to entertain your baby, just make sure that it is safe. This is especially important as soon as your baby starts to move about more and then to reach out for things. So for example if you tie something to the cot, make sure there is no way your baby could get twisted or tangled up in the string or ribbon. Likewise, when the baby begins to crawl make sure that there are no uncovered electric sockets where the baby could push his finger.

Bringing up a baby requires much patience and love and affection. A baby needs to be held and soothed when he is disturbed or hurt and you must treat him at all times with respect and understanding. A happy and contented baby will generally grow into a good-natured, secure and a loving individual who has confidence in self. All parents yearn for these qualities in their children, but few realise the mistakes they often make while raising their child. A good beginning is a must for a bright and sunny future –your efforts must be guided by this basic thought!

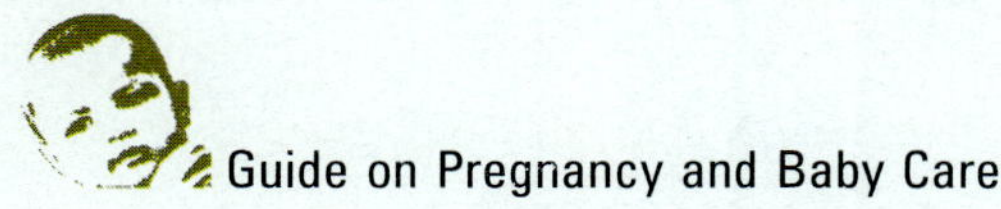

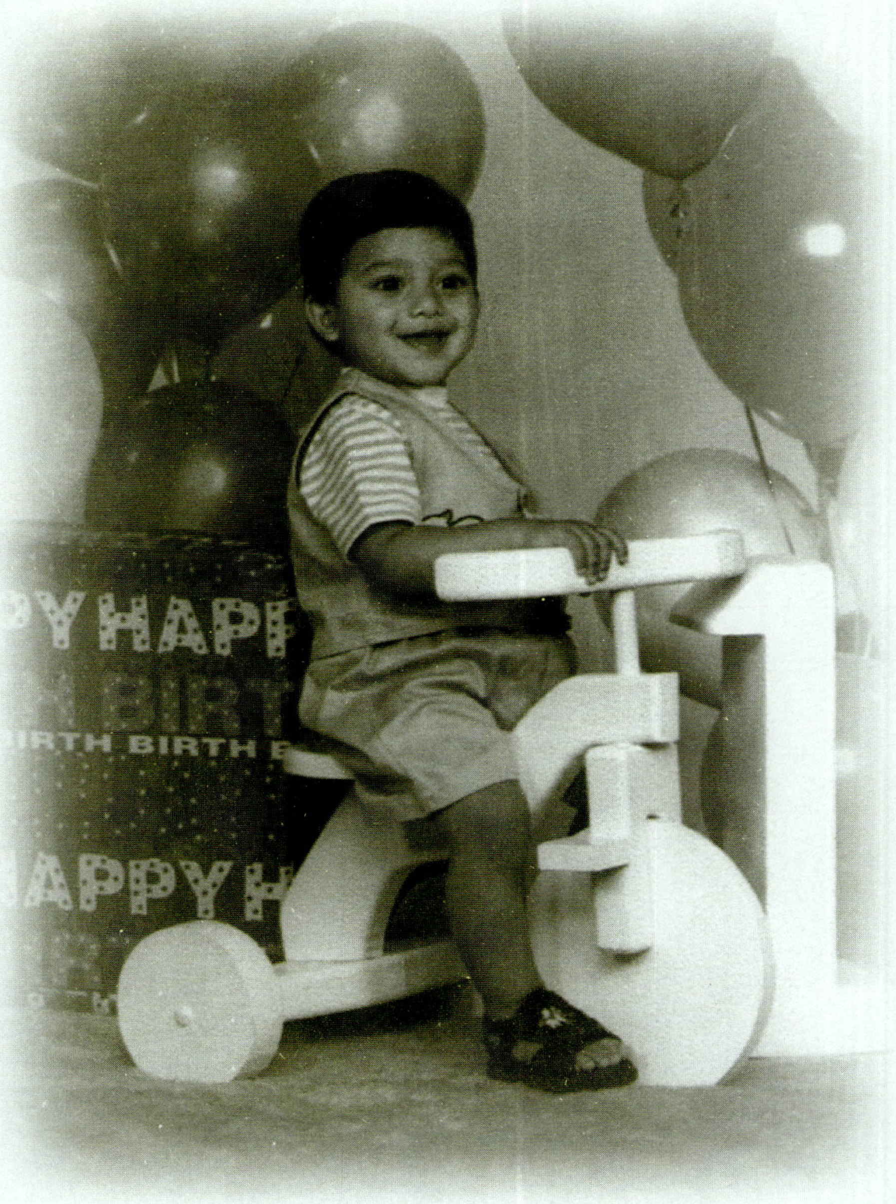

Appendices

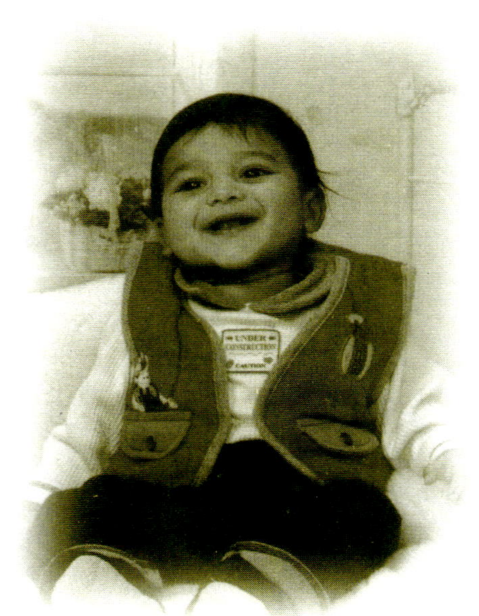

Maternity Benefits

Maternity leave

1. Admissible to married/unmarried women employees during-
   (a). Pregnancy: 135 days. Admissible only to employees with less than two surviving children. Rule 43 (1).
   (b). Miscarriage/ abortion (induced or otherwise): Total of 45 days in the entire service excluding any such leave taken prior to 16.6.1994. Admissible irrespective of number of surviving children. Application should be supported by a certificate from a Registered Medical Practitioner for non-governmental organisations and from an authorised medical attendant for governmental organisations. Rule 43 (3).
2. The leave is not debited to the leave account. Rule 43 (5).
3. It is granted on full pay. Rule 43 (2).
4. The leave may be combined with leave of any other kind. Rule 43 (4).
5. Any leave (including commuted leave up to 60 days and leave not due) may be taken without medical certificate up to one year in continuation. Rule 43 (4).
6. Counts as service for increments. FR 26(b).
7. Counts as service for pension. Rule 21 of CCS (Pension) Rules.
8. In the case of officials to whom the provisions of Employees' State Insurance Act apply, the leave salary will be reduced by the benefit admissible under the Act for corresponding period. Note below Rule 43 (2).
9. Not admissible for 'threatened abortion'. GID (4), Rule 43.

Paternity Leave

Eligibility: Male government servants with less than two surviving children. Apprentices are also eligible.
Duration: 15 days during the wife's confinement.
Leave Salary: Equal to last pay drawn.
Not to be debited to the leave account. May be combined with any other kind of leave except casual leave.
Not to be refused normally. O.M. dated 7.10. 1997
To be applied up to 15 days before or up to six months from date of delivery. O.M. dated 16.7.1999

The Calorie Count

Foods and beverages	Amount or Average Serving	Calorie Count
Breads		
Phulka	One	85
Paratha	One	150
Aloo Ka Paratha	One	213
Puri	One	80
Pathura	One	154
Bread	1 slice	60
Hamburger on bun	3-inch patty	500
Rice [Ready to serve]		
Rice	2 katori	222
Pulao	2 katori	358
Kicheri	2 katori	430

Dal (Ready to serve)		
Moong ki Dal	1 katori	116
Arhar ki dal	1 katori	109
Masoor ki dal	1 katori	148
Urd ki dal	1 katori	161
Samber	1 katori	81
Kabuli Chana	1 katori	119
Saboot Moong ki dal	1 katori	113
Rajma	1 katori	153
Vegetarian delicacies		
Preparations with gravy		
Matar Paneer	1 katori	191
Aloo Matar	1 katori	132
Aloo ki sabzi	1 katori	130
Vegetable kofta	1 katori	217
Vegetable korma	1 katori	132
Dry preparations		
Aloo baingan	1 katori	134
Aloo shimla mirch	1 katori	116
Bhindi	1 katori	150
Parmal	1 katori	78
Torai	1 katori	97
Seetaphal	1 katori	110
Bhurtha	1 katori	152
Patta gobhi (cabbage)	1 katori	131
Stuffed tomato	1 no.	84
Vegetable cutlets	2 nos	132
Mixed vegetable	1 katori	100

Non-Vegetarian delicacies		
Tandoori Chicken	125g	257
Fish Cutlets	2 nos.	190
Mutton Curry	6 pieces	237
Liver do piazza	140 g	330
Prawn curry	145 g	219
Fruits		
Apple	One 3-inch	90
Banana	One 6-inch	100
Grapes	30 medium	75
Orange	One 2¾-inch	80
Pear	One	100
Mango	One medium	180
Desserts & Sweets		
Jelly and Custard	One katori	104
Kheer	One katori	332
Savian	One katori	249
Suji ki kheer	One katori	267
Srikand	½ katori	382
Gulab jamun	Two pieces	387
Sandesh	Two pieces	140
Jalebi	100 gm	494
Cake		
2 layers, iced white	One serving	345
Fruit, 1/4 –inch slice		125
Ice Creams		
Chocolate	Small cup	150
Vanilla, strawberry	Small cup	130
Sundaes	Average	400

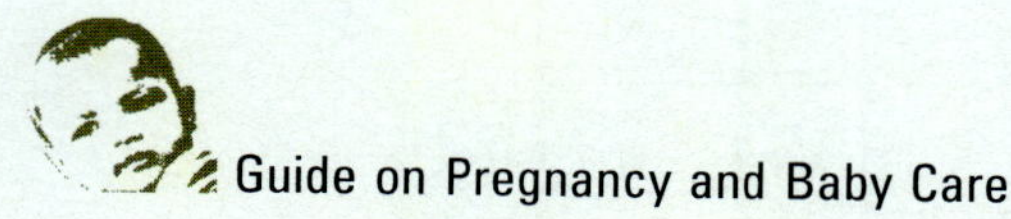

Ice cream sodas, chocolate	300 ml.	270
Chocolate bars		
Plain	One bar	190
With nuts	(35 gm.)	278
Snacks		
Pakoras	8 pieces	280
Basen ka pura	one	222
Dahi vada	Two pieces	343
Vada	Two pieces	138
Masala Dosa	One	205
Cocconut Dosa	One	312
Onion Dosa	One	409
Idli	Two	132
Kachori	Two	383
Aloo ka Bonda	Two	200
Samosa	One	207
Pizza, cheese	One	1440
Potato chips	One serving	108
Beverages		
Cola beverages	300ml.	140
Carbonated beverages	200ml.	100
Tea or coffee, no cream or sugar	One cup	0
Tea or coffee, 2 tbsp cream 2tsf sugar	One cup	90
Hot Chocolate	One cup	200
Salted nuts		
Almonds	10	130
Cashews	10	60
Peanuts	10	60

Glossary

Abortion: Expulsion of the embryo or foetus from the uterus before it becomes viable. Even though modern neonatology centres endeavour to lower this age, it is taken as any time before the 28th week after conception. Spontaneous abortion, or miscarriage, may be caused by death of the foetus due to a genetic abnormality in the fertilised egg, its inability to find a proper place for itself in the uterus or a infection or disease in the expectant mother. Abortion may also be induced, the foetus removed from the uterus by such methods as vacuum suction, dilation and curettage, intra-uterine saline injection and surgically opening the uterus (hysterectomy).

By general agreement, accidental or spontaneous cases are referred to as miscarriages and deliberately induced ones as abortions.

Accoucheur: Obstetrician; specialist in midwifery.

Albumin: The most abundant of the proteins dissolved in blood.

Anaemia: Literally, anaemia means lack of blood, but in fact it is shortage of haemoglobin, the oxygen-carrying pigment of the red blood cells. The effects of anaemia are due to shortage of oxygen throughout the body.

Antepartum: Before childbirth.

Antepartum haemorrhage: bleeding from the uterus before delivery of the child, commonly because the placenta lies below the baby and becomes dislodged before labour set in. At times, disruption of the placenta from the uterine wall can also lead to such bleeding.

Antibiotic: A class of drug used to treat infection. Biologists of the 19th century knew that one type of microbe might oppose the growth of another. This antagonism is called antibiosis. The first antibiotics were produced using this very principle, with the help of one mould or bacterium; but later synthetic analogue antibiotics were also developed.

Antiseptic: Chemical used to destroy microbes.

Areola: Pigmented skin around the nipple.

BCG (bacille Calmette-Guerin): A vaccine against tuberculosis, prepared from a strain of bacilli that have lost their virulence after years of growth in an artificial medium. It was first prepared at the Pasteur Institute in Paris in 1906 by Leon Calmette and Camille Guerin and used to prevent tuberculosis. It has been used for human vaccination since 1922, but its value has always been thought to be doubtful.

Birthmark: A congenital blemish of the skin, of which there are several types. Birthmarks include the pigmented nevus or mole, which is a conglomeration of pigment cells resembling those scattered throughout the skin, and several types of vascular nevus composed of small blood vessels. Unless there are very strong cosmetic reasons for interfering, most birthmarks are best left alone.

Bladder: The bladder is a flexible muscular bag. It receives a continuous dribble of urine from the kidneys, which it empties out from time to time.

Blood groups: A red blood cell has a thin shell, of which the chemical structure differs slightly in different people. Several components of the shell vary. A component and its variants form a system. People whose red cells have the same variant belong to the same blood group as regards that particular system.

At least 14 systems have been described. Since they are independent of each other there are many possible combinations. The great importance of blood groups in medicine is that chemical compounds different from those of an individual are treated as 'foreign' by his body defences. If red cells of a foreign group enter his blood, they are liable to be destroyed as though they were infecting bacteria.

Karl Landsteiner, in Vienna, discovered the most important of the blood-group systems, the ABO system, in 1900. 'Blood group' normally means the ABO group (A, B, AB, or 0). Rhesus factor is the basis of the other major system of blood groups and was discovered in 1940, again by Landsteiner. Some dangerous illnesses of newborn babies are due to their belonging to a different rhesus group from their mothers.

Blood pressure (BP): The pressure at which the heart pumps blood into the major arteries. Subject to some individual variation, a normal BP fluctuates with the heartbeat between about 120 mm of mercury (systolic pressure), and 80 mm (diastolic pressure).

Breech = Buttocks.

Breech delivery: The birth of a baby buttocks-first, instead of the usual head-first. It adds to the difficulties of both mother and child, and is usually avoided by turning the baby to a head-down position before confinement. When breech delivery cannot be avoided, it is facilitated by bringing the baby's feet down so that the baby's legs are born straight and not bunched in front of his belly.

Caesarean section: Surgical operation, at a late stage of pregnancy. The abdominal wall is opened and the incision is carried through the front of the uterus, the baby is lifted out, and the layers of the incision are stitched. Caesarean section is used when the birthpassage is too narrow for the baby, or when the placenta lies across the passage from the uterus and would be liable to bleed dangerously during natural labour, or in any situation where the health of mother or infant requires immediate delivery.

Candida (Monilia): A fungus related to the yeasts.

Carotene: Orange pigment of carrots and many other vegetables also found in egg yolk and milk; converted in the body to vitamin A.

Cell: The smallest unit of the body that is capable of independent life. The whole body is a community of individual cells of which the primary function is to maintain a suitable environment for themselves and for each other.

Cervix: Neck of the womb; the part of the uterus that projects into the upper part of the vagina. It is a powerful ring of muscle, closed at most times but able to expand widely during childbirth.

Cloning: To reproduce or propagate asexually by making multiple identical copies of a DNA sequence and thus maintaining a pure lineage of a cell under laboratory conditions.

Cramp: Painful spasm (sustained contraction) of muscles.

Cystitis: Inflammation of the urinary bladder, usually from bacterial infection.

Diabetes mellitus: Diabetes mellitus, or simply diabetes, is the result of a deficiency of insulin, a hormone secreted by the pancreas to regulate the use of sugar (glucose). The deficiency can be caused in more than one way. The effects are far-reaching. The most obvious and least important are: excess of glucose in the blood (which is quite harmless), overflow of glucose into the urine, and increased volume of urine to carry the glucose. This increased volume of urine leads to increased thirst, which may be the first symptom of diabetes.

Diagnosis: The identification or recognition of diseases. Apart from a few cases where the culprit practically gives itself up, it is a process or elimination from a group of suspects, starting with the premise that anyone might have any conceivable disease.

Diaphragm: Sheet of muscle separating the thorax from the abdomen. Its fibres arise from the lumbar vertebrae, the lower ribs, and the lower end of the sternum. They converge on a flat sheet of dense fibrous tissue, the central tendon. The whole structure forms a sort of dome. When the muscle contracts, the central tendon is pulled down, the thorax is enlarged, and air is drawn into the lungs to fill the extra space. This is the most important mechanical factor in respiration.

Dilatation = Widening or stretching.

Drug: In non-technical language, drug has come to suggest a narcotic or habit-forming substance. In the technical sense, a drug is any substance taken medicinally to help recovery from sickness or relieve symptoms, or to modify any natural process in the body.

Eclampsia: Convulsions occurring at the end of pregnancy as a result of toxaemia.

Ectopic: In an abnormal anatomical situation. Ectopic pregnancy occurs when a fertilized ovum, instead of passing down the Fallopian tube and implanting itself in the lining of the uterus, settles in the tube or elsewhere. Such a pregnancy seldom lasts more than 2 or 3 months, though cases have been reported in which an infant has survived in the cavity of the abdomen for long enough to be born live by Caesarean section. In most cases the embryo dies early and is absorbed. Occasionally the Fallopian tube bursts and bleeds, and an immediate operation is needed to repair the damage.

Embryo: An organism in its early stages of development, especially before it has reached a distinctively recognisable form. In human biology: an unborn offspring from the time of fertilisation until the first two months of pregnancy.

Endoderm: A layer of cells at a very early stage in the development of an embryo, the inner of the three germ layers. The digestive organs and lungs are derived from it.

Endometrium: The lining of the womb.

Epididymis: Organ at the top of the testicle where sperms are stored.

Epilepsy: An ill-defined group of disorders characterized by fits (seizures). A fit is an episode of disorganized and excessive activity in some part of the brain, causing disturbances of sensation, movement or consciousness according to the area of the brain that is involved.

Erythrocyte = red blood cell.

Erythrocyte sedimentation rate (ESR): is a clinical laboratory test. It is the rate at which the red cells settle in a column of blood in a glass tube. Rapid sedimentation suggests that the disease under investigation is still active.

Fallopian tubes: A pair of tubes open at one end to the cavity of the abdomen and at the other to the upper part of the uterus. The abdominal end, which looks not unlike a sea anemone, is next to the ovary. It collects the ovum that is shed each month and conveys it to the uterus. Sperms swim up the tubes from the uterus, and fertilisation takes place in the Fallopian tube; the fertilised ovum begins to develop into an embryo before it reaches the uterus.

Fertilisation: The meeting of sperm with a ripe egg cell.

Foetus: Unborn infant that has developed from an embryo to a stage where it is recognisably human, i.e. from about the ninth week of pregnancy.

Folic acid: A vitamin of the B group present in all green plants.

Follicle Stimulating Hormone (FSH): A hormone released by the pituitary gland, which stimulates one or more follicles in the ovary to mature.

Forceps, obstetric: Tongs ending in curved loops, shaped to hold a baby's head firmly but safely; used to ease the head past a resistant outlet when birth is delayed at the final stage; invented in about 1600 by an English obstetrician, Peter Chamberlen.

Gamete: A sex cell, either ovum or sperm.

German measles (rubella): A very common virus infection in childhood, with slight fever, swollen lymph nodes, and a characteristic rash. It is a much milder illness than true measles. After an incubation of two to three weeks, the attack starts with headache, fretfulness and a rising temperature, followed a day later by a pink rash spreading from the face. Lymph nodes–typically, behind the ears–are enlarged and sore. The symptoms seldom last more than 3 or 4 days. The patient is infectious from the day before symptoms begin until the day after they disappear. German measles was thought unimportant until it was shown to injure embryos.

Until the third month of pregnancy, the developing infant does not resist the virus. Instead, the virus is accepted as though it were part of the natural chemical composition of the embryo and allowed to multiply freely. The result is that numerous organs grow abnormally. The effect may be so serious that the embryo simply dies and is aborted; but some of these infants (still carrying the live virus 6 or 7 months after infection) are born with serious defects. In the opinion of many competent people the risk justifies artificial abortion after German measles in early pregnancy. It is clearly in the interests of girls to take the vaccine against this disease before they marry.

Gestation: The duration of pregnancy. Human gestation lasts on average 38 weeks from conception to confinement, but is more easily measured from the beginning of the last menstrual period as 40 weeks.

Glucose: A simple sugar, its combustion with oxygen to form water and carbon dioxide is the principal source of energy in the body. Even without oxygen, some energy is got by converting glucose to lactic acid. Food contains little if any glucose as such, but all starch and sugar in the diet is changed to glucose by digestion.

Gonads: The primary sex organs; ovaries in women and testes in men.

Haemoglobin: The red pigment of the blood, carried by the red blood cells. It is composed of a protein, globin, and an iron compound, haem. It is the means of transporting oxygen from the lungs to the rest of the body.

Haemorrhoids (piles): Distended (varicose) veins at the junction of rectum and anal canal, about an inch above the opening of the anus.

Herpes: Two quite different virus infections are known as herpes.

Herpes simplex is a clutch of inflamed blisters ('cold sore') around the mouth or occasionally some other mucous membrane. Most people carry the virus all their lives, without symptoms. A few develop blisters when they have some other infection; exposure to very hot or very cold weather may also cause an eruption. Apart from rare cases of serious infection in infants, this is a harmless disorder.

Herpes zoster is caused by the same virus as chickenpox. The virus, like that of herpes simplex, lies dormant in the tissues and may flare up many years after the chickenpox. The virus establishes itself around sensory nerve cells about to enter the spinal cord, and causes painful blisters in the area of skin served by the affected nerves.

Hormone: A substance released into the bloodstream by one organ to regulate the function of others.

Hyaline membrane disease= Respiratory distress syndrome, a common cause of death among newborn babies. The baby is born alive, and usually starts to breath, but cannot keep his lungs filled with air. Unless breathing can be maintained artificially the baby asphyxiates and dies.

Hydrocephalus: Enlargement of an infant's head by accumulation of cerebrospinal fluid, due to blockage of its normal circulation in and around the brain and spinal cord. Various surgical operations have been devised to relieve the pressure and prevent damage to the brain.

Hypertension=High blood pressure.

Hypoglycaemia=Deficiency of sugar in the blood.

Icterus=jaundice. This occurs when bilirubin, a reddish-yellow bile pigment in the body, becomes abnormally high.

Immunisation: Production of immunity to an infectious disease by artificial means, i.e. other than by an attack of the disease itself. Vaccination, the oldest established method of immunisation, is the injection of live microbes, so modified that they are practically harmless yet still induce immunity.

Implantation: When a fertilised egg becomes fixed in the wall of the uterus. This occurs about six days after conception.

Induction: Induction of labour is the use of artificial means to start the process of childbirth if there has been undue delay or the health of mother or child is at risk. The hospital routine of warm bath followed by enema, followed if necessary by injections of oxytocin, a pituitary hormone, to stimulate the uterus, often works. If this fails, releasing a little fluid from the membranous bag surrounding the baby may set off contractions of the uterus. Successful induction may avoid Caesarean section.

Labour: The process by which a pregnant woman is delivered of her baby.

Lumbar: The part of the back between the lowest pair of ribs and the top of the pelvis. This includes the five lumbar vertebrae.

Luteinising hormone: A hormone released by the anterior part of the pituitary gland, the surge of which in mid menstrual cycle leads to the egg release.

Meconium: Greenish fluid, mostly bile and mucus, in an infant's intestine, passed soon after birth, or before birth if labour is difficult and the infant is distressed.

Menstruation: Periodic bleeding in women of childbearing age.

Monilia => Thrush

Mongol (mongoloid): Affected with mongolism or Down's syndrome, a defect of growth due to a fault in the formation of the ovum. Normally the fertilised ovum receives one member of each pair of chromosomes from each parent, but a faulty germ cell may contribute two chromosomes of the same type, and the embryo then gets three instead of a pair. This particular defect occurs in relation to chromosome 21. Growth and mental development are retarded, and among other physical peculiarities the child develops features vaguely suggestive of a Mongolian. The defect is common occurring in one in 700 live births. Mongols are friendly and cheerful, and although they need special education they can generally look after themselves and learn to occupy themselves usefully.

Obstetrician: Specialist in the management of childbirth.

Obstetrics: Midwifery; medical care in pregnancy and childbirth.

Oestrogen: A steroid hormone produced chiefly by the ovaries and responsible for promoting oestrus and the development and maintenance of a woman's secondary sex characteristics.

Ovaries: Two small almond shaped organs at either side of the uterus where eggs are produced.

Ovum (plural ova): Latin for egg. An ovum is released from the ovary once a mouth.

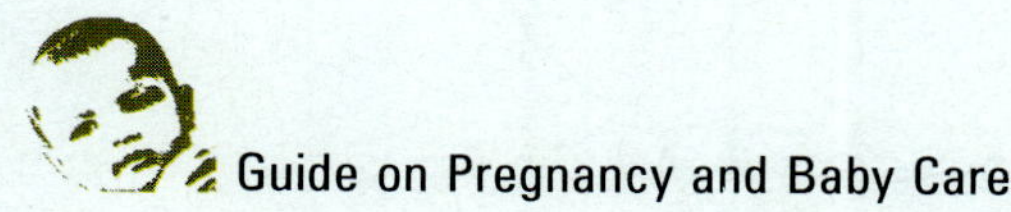

Oxytocin. A hormone released from the posterior lobe of the pituitary gland. It stimulates the contraction of smooth muscle of the uterus during labour and facilitates ejection of milk from the breast during nursing.

Paracetamol: A medicine used to find relief from fever and pain and considered to be very safe.

Pituitary gland: A small, oval endocrine gland situated at the base of the brain. It is called the master gland because the other endocrine glands depend on its secretions for stimulation. The pituitary has two distinct lobes, anterior and posterior. The gonadotropin hormones, which stimulate the ovaries in a female and testes in males, are formed in its anterior lobe.

Pelvis: Lower limb-girdle, composed of the lower part of the backbone and the two hipbones. The pelvis is a firm ring of bone. The centrepiece is the sacrum, consisting of five vertebrae fused into a single bone, broad and massive in its upper part and tapering to a point below, to which the rudimentary tail (coccyx) is attached. The hipbones (haunches) are attached to either side of the sacrum at the rigid sacroiliac joints. In front the hipbones meet at the symphysis pubis, where they are bound together with tough fibrous tissue. In the male, these joints are practically rigid; in the female they allow slight adjustment of the pelvis during childbirth.

Deformity of the pelvis, however slight, is important to women because it may cause difficulty with childbirth, even a normal pelvis leaves little room to spare. The so-called contracted pelvis is not deformed but simply the relatively small pelvis of a woman with small bones, which may cause trouble if she has a large baby. A more real and serious deformity is caused by rickets in childhood, or any other illness that interferes with the growth of bones. In all these cases, Caesarean section solves the problem.

Penis: Male copulatory organ. The penis is constructed of three columns of erectile stissue: the two corpora cavernosa placed side by side, and the corpus spongiosum below them. The end of the corpus spongiosum is enlarged to form the conical tip (glans penis). Erectile tissue consists mainly of a labyrinth of blood vessels.

Erection is simply distension of the tissue with blood: the veins are compressed by reflex contraction of muscle fibres around them while the arteries are dilated. The urethra, a tube for the passage of urine or semen, traverses the corpus spongiosum. The muscles that close the veins during erection also close the outlet from the urinary bladder.

Perinatal: The period shortly before, during and shortly after birth. This period is taken from the 28th week of pregnancy until the infant is a month old.

Perineum: The external aspect of the outlet of the pelvis, i.e. the region enclosed by the thighs and the lower part of the buttocks, including the external genital organs and the anal canal. The term is often—especially in obstetrics—used to describe the bridge of muscle and fibrous tissue between the genital organs and the anus, which is very liable to be injured during childbirth.

Pessary: Soluble gelatinous preparation for introducing antiseptic or other drugs into the vagina; vaginal suppository.

Phocomelia: A grave congenital defect of the limbs: the hands and feet are fairly normal, but the arms and legs fail to grow. The hands and feet spring from the shoulders and hips like the flippers of a seal. This rare deformity suddenly became much commoner when the drug, thalidomide, was on the market.

Placenta: Organ by which an unborn infant gets nourishment from its mother. The placenta develops from the layer of cells surrounding those destined to form the body itself. It is a part of the growing infant's tissues, not the mother's, and its dense network of blood vessels communicates by way of the umbilical vein and arteries with the circulation of the infant. The placenta is firmly attached to the lining of the mother's uterus, but no blood passes between the two. Dissolved oxygen and nutrients diffuse from the mother's blood to the placenta, and carbon dioxide and other waste products diffuse in the opposite direction. The placenta is released shortly after the birth of the infant, to whom it is still joined by the umbilical cord. At this stage it forms a thick disc, some 15 cm across, weighing 400 grams.

In addition to its main functions as an organ of respiration, nutrition, and excretion for the infant, the placenta acts as an endocrine gland for the mother, secreting hormones that diffuse into her circulation and maintain pregnancy till the 20th week.

Placenta praevia: An unusual situation of the placenta, which lies across the opening of the uterus instead of high up and out of the way during birth. It is a cause of bleeding before or during labour, and may necessitate Caesarean section.

Postmaturity: Condition of an infant at birth after unduly prolonged pregnancy. If labour is delayed beyond a week or two after the normal time for pregnancy to end, the risk to the child may be almost as great as that of prematurity, because the placenta is no longer able to nourish the child sufficiently. The mother's difficulties may be increased if the child's bones begin to harden. Postmaturity is treated either by artificial induction of labour, or by Caesarean section.

Prolactin: Lactogenic hormone, formed in the anterior lobe of the pituitary and stimulating the formation of milk.

Prolapse: Displacement of an organ from its normal position, usually by gravity as a result of weakness of the supporting tissues.

Progesterone: A hormone secreted by the corpus luteum, i.e. the small gland that develops in an ovary each month at the site from which an ovum or egg has been released. Progesterone stimulates development of the uterus to receive a fertilised ovum and nourish the embryo. If the ovum is fertilised and pregnancy occurs, the corpus luteum and later the placenta continue to form progesterone, which prevents menstruation and the release of more ova. If pregnancy does not occur, the corpus luteum withers. The action of progesterone in preventing ova from being shed is the basis of the contraceptive pill.

Pseudocyesis: False pregnancy, with symptoms of a real pregnancy. The basis is emotional, but emotion affects the formation of hormones by the pituitary gland, with physical effects like those of pregnancy.

Prostate gland: A gland in men surrounding the urethra at the base of the bladder. It secretes a fluid which is a major constituent of semen.

Puberty: Onset of sexual maturity or fertility, brought about by stimulation of the gonads (ovaries or testicles) by hormones from the pituitary gland. The gonads begin to form fertile ova or sperms, and also to secrete hormones that promote adult sexual characters.

Puerperal: Related to childbirth; affecting a woman who bas recently given birth. Puerperal fever (puerperal pyrexia) can mean any high temperature following childbirth, but is generally taken to mean infection of the birth passage as a result of childbirth.

Rickets: Faulty growth of bone, due to lack of vitamin D. The vitamin is formed in human skin exposed to sunlight. Children deprived of sunlight need vitamin D in their diet (fish, milk, eggs). Rickets affects those who cannot find the vitamin from either source. The net result of this deficiency is that calcium salts are not deposited in sufficient amount in the bone to make it rigid. The cartilage at the growing ends of long bones is enlarged, e.g. at the front ends of the ribs and at the knees; and weight-bearing bones are twisted out of shape. Women affected with rickets often need assistance during childbirth.

Rubella = German measles.

Scrotum: A loose bag of skin containing the testes, which function at a few degrees below the temperature of the rest of the body.

Scurvy: A defect of the substance that binds cells together, especially in connective tissue and capillary blood vessels, due to lack of vitamin C. The usual cause is lack of fresh vegetables or fruit; but healing of severe injuries or inflammation makes heavy demands on the supply of vitamin C and may cause a relative deficiency even with an average diet. The symptoms include bleeding into the skin, around bones, into joints, and from the gums. The teeth become loose and misshapen. Resistance to infection is lowered.

Seminal vesicles: A pair of pouch like glands situated on each side of the male urinary bladder that secrete seminal fluid and nourish and promote the movement of spermatozoa through the urethra.

Shock: Failure of the circulation of blood when the blood pressure is too low to maintain an adequate flow through the tissues and back to the heart.

Spermatozoon (sperm): The male reproductive cells.

Syphilis: A sexually transmitted disease caused by the bacteria Treponema pallidum.

Testicle (testis): Like its counterpart the ovary, the testis has two distinct functions. It forms the male germ cells, sperms; and it is also an endocrine gland, secreting sex hormones into the bloodstream.

Testosterone: The male sex hormone that is produced in the testis.

Tetanus: Spasm of voluntary muscles with convulsions, caused by infection with the tetanus bacillus, Clostridium tetani. Lack of hygiene during childbirth can lead to this serious infection.

Tetracycline: An antibiotic prepared from chlortetracycline, which is extracted from the fungus Streptomyces aureofaciens. It should not be used by a pregnant mother.

Thalidomide: Sedative drug first used in Germany in 1958, and withdrawn in 1961 because of serious deformities among babies born to women who had taken the drug during pregnancy.

Thrush (Candidiasis): A common vaginal infection, which can develop without sexual contact. It usually only affects females and can be easily cleared up with anti fungal agents.

Toxaemia (of pregnancy): A serious ailment that affects some women during pregnancy and disappears as soon as the pregnancy is over. The symptoms are accumulation of water in the tissues, first noticed as undue swelling of the ankles; loss of protein in the urine; and high blood pressure.

Trichomoniasis: A vaginal inflammation caused by protozoa, Trichomonas vaginalis. It often causes a refractory discharge and itching.

Twins: Fraternal (dizygotic, binovular) twins develop when two ova are fertilised at the same time. As a rule a woman's ovaries release only a single ovum each month, but if two or more happen to be released together they can be fertilised together. A tendency to shed more than one ovum can be inherited, so that fraternal twins occur more often in some families than others. If pituitary hormones or the synthetic drug clomiphene are used to stimulate the ovaries (for treatment of infertility), then several ova can be released all at once.

Identical (monozygotic, monovular) twins develop from the two halves of a single ovum, formed as the first step in the growth of an embryo.

About one pregnancy in 90 produces twins; and according to Hellin's law one in 8100 produces triplets and one in 7,29,000 quadruplets

Ultrasound: Vibrations of the same kind as sound waves, but of such high frequency that they cannot be heard. Extremely useful as a diagnosis tool, and being very safe, they are today routinely used to check the growing baby in mother's womb.

Umbilical cord: A bundle of two arteries and a vein, surrounded by a clear gelatinous material and a thin membrane, connecting an unborn infant with its placenta. The cord is normally sealed with a ligature and cut soon after birth, and the remaining stump withers and falls off.

Urethra: The tube that carries urine from the bladder to the outside of the body.

Uterus (womb): A hollow muscular organ located in the pelvic cavity of women in which the fertilised egg implants and develops.

Vaccine: A virus or bacterium so modified (e.g. by culture in an unnatural environment or treatment with formaldehyde) as to be no longer dangerous, yet able to confer immunity in the same way as infection with the actual disease.

Vagina: The passage leading from the opening of the vulva to the cervix of the uterus in women.

Valve: Several tubes inside the body are provided with valves. They restrict flow to one direction.

Vas deferens: The main duct through which semen is carried from the epididymis to the ejaculatory duct.

Venereal disease: Infectious disease usually transmitted by sexual contact. The common ones are gonorrhoea and syphilis, which are both caused by bacteria and are treatable with suitable antibiotics, and the killer viral disease, AIDS.

Vulva: The external female genitals.

Zygote: Cell produced by fusion of male and female germ cells; fertilised ovum.

Further Reading

- Agarwal, Yatish: Bodytalk—The Good Health Guide, First Edition (2000). Rupa & Co., New Delhi.
- Daftary, S. N. and Chakravarti, S. (ed.) : Holland and Brews Manual of Obstetrics, Sixth Edition (1998). B I Churchill Livingstone, New Delhi.
- Dutta, D.C.: Text Book of Obstetrics, Third Edition (1995). New Central Book Agency (P) Ltd., Kolkata.
- Ghai, O.P.: Essential Paediatrics, Fourth Edition (1996). Interprint, New Delhi.
- Indian Council of Medical Research: Nutritional Requirements and Recommended Dietary Allowances for Indians (1998). New Delhi.
- Krishna Menon M.K. and Palaniappan B. (ed): Mudaliar and Menon's Clinical Obstetrics, Ninth edition (1994). Orient Longman Limited, Hyderabad.
- Ministry of Health and Family Welfare, Government of India: Annual Report 1999-2000. Government of India Press.
- Park, K. (ed): Park's Textbook of Preventive and Social Medicine, Fifteenth Edition (1998). Banarasidas Bhanot Publishers, Jabalpur.